SILENT RUNNING

OUR FAMILY'S JOURNEY TO THE FINISH LINE WITH AUTISM

Robyn K. Schneider
with Kate Hopper

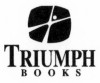

TRIUMPH
BOOKS

Library of Congress Cataloging-in-Publication Data

Schneider, Robyn K.
Silent running: our family's journey to the finish line with autism / Robyn K. Schneider; with Kate Hopper.
    pages cm
ISBN 978-1-62937-091-0 (hardback)
    1. Schneider, Robyn K. 2. Schneider, Alex, 1990—Mental health. 3. Schneider, Jamie, 1990—Mental health. 4. Autistic children—New York (State)—Long Island—Biography. 5. Autistic children—Rehabilitation—New York (State)—Long Island. 6. Autistic children—Family relationships—New York (State)—Long Island. 7. Parents of autistic children—New York (State)—Long Island—Biography. 8. Running—Therapeutic use—New York (State)—Long Island. I. Title.
    RJ506.A9S389 2015
    618.92'858820092—dc23
    [B]
                                                          2014048219

This book is available in quantity at special discounts for your group or organization. For further information, contact:

Triumph Books LLC
814 North Franklin Street
Chicago, Illinois 60610
(312) 337-0747
www.triumphbooks.com

Printed in U.S.A.
ISBN: 978-1-62937-091-0
Design by Patricia Frey
Page production by Alex Lubertozzi
Photos courtesy of Robyn K. Schneider

*In memory of my beloved parents,
Frances and Ingram, whose enduring and unconditional love
remains deep within my heart.*

*To my sons, Alex and Jamie. You have given me infinite joy
and love, and I treasure you each and every day.*

So many of our dreams at first seem impossible,
then they seem improbable,
and then, when we summon the will,
they soon become inevitable.

—*Christopher Reeve*

Author's Note

This is a work of memory, and though memory is flawed, I have tried to be truthful and, where possible, verify my memories using records from the past, research, and through conversation with those who are in my story. Names and other identifying characteristics of some people have been changed or omitted to protect their identities.

Prologue

THE EARLY MORNING AIR is chilly, but the sun is bright—the perfect day for a marathon. I make my way into the throng of people at the starting line to kiss my son Jamie and squeeze my husband, Allan's, arm. Jamie smiles, though his eyes are searching the sky above the crowd. Allan gives me a quick hug. I know he's nervous.

"Good luck! I love you," I say. And then, fighting back tears, I add, "Have a great run!"

I move forward until I can see my other son Alex, Jamie's identical twin. Alex's coach, Kevin, is next to him, and they're near the front, flanked by the elites. I know Kevin is anxious, as well. The boys only train three days a week, and Kevin says you can fake a short race on three days, but a marathon is a whole different game. Alex—Alie— is looking straight ahead, a huge smile on his face. Even if he doesn't know that he's running his first marathon, he knows it's a race day, and his joy is almost palpable. Unlike the runners surrounding him, he's not worried about his time. He doesn't have a plan. He just knows he gets to run.

Still, I can't help but feel apprehensive. Alie had a rough morning, and I'm worried it will affect his race. What if something on the course sets him off again? But he looks calm now. I give myself a mental shake. He's ready.

I shiver as I watch the other runners pull one foot and then another up behind them, stretching their quads. They glance down at their watches, adjust their race numbers, and pull their arms across their chests, stretching their shoulders.

The boys are 20 years old, and this is their 70th race, so I shouldn't be as nervous as I am. But it's their first marathon, and I'm worried. What if something goes wrong? What if one of them gets hurt? Or worse, lost?

I find my friends Randy and Leslie in the crowd. Leslie, who is married to Kevin, is holding their five-year-old daughter Mercy on her hip. Mercy is smiling widely, taking in the music and the people. I wish I could give myself over to the thrill of the moment, too, but instead I grab Randy's arm. "Do you think they're going to be okay?"

Randy is a marathoner and has known the boys since they were toddlers. She was the one who first encouraged us to get them into running, and she's giddy with excitement. "They're going to do great!" she laughs, tucking her dark curly hair behind her ear.

Leslie smiles and says the same thing. "They've worked so hard for this."

Yesterday we drove the two hours from our home in Great Neck, Long Island, to the Hamptons, picked up the race packets, and had a big pasta dinner with Randy, Kevin, Leslie, and Mercy. The boys were all smiles during dinner, familiar with the ritual of carbo-loading the night before a big race. Back at our hotel, they watched me lay out their running clothes on the couch, pinning their race numbers to their shirts. I knew they were happy; there were huge smiles frozen on their narrow faces. I wondered, as I had thousands of times, what they were thinking. What was going through their minds?

When I was done laying everything out, Alie smoothed each item of clothing with his hands until all the wrinkles had been eliminated. Then he arranged all of our running shoes—mine, Allan's, his own, and Jamie's—in an arcing horseshoe on the floor, the laces of every shoe pulled taut to each side, the tip of one lace just barely touching the tip of the next one. Allan and I smiled, shaking our heads.

Now Kevin is holding Alie's hand, as he always does at the starting line, and they've moved to the front of the pack. Kevin and Alie have been running together for four years now, and I wouldn't have Alie run this race with anyone else.

I take a deep breath, and my eyes fill with tears as I think about what Kevin said before a race a few years ago: tomorrow morning all the runners will return to their normal busy lives—commuting to work and going to school—and Alie and Jamie will be at a distinct disadvantage. But today when that gun goes off, it's a level playing field. Today, they're just runners.

1

ALIE AND JAMIE were happy babies. They smiled easily and loved to laugh. When I think back on their first year, I see a photograph Allan took when they were newborns: I'm sitting on the couch in our two-bedroom apartment wearing a T-shirt and shorts. I'm a little disheveled, my light brown hair pulled into a messy ponytail. Both boys are in my lap side by side, their tiny heads resting on my left arm. My left hand reaches around to give Jamie his bottle and my right hand holds Alie's bottle.

It wasn't easy—or comfortable—but to me it was the most natural thing in the world. I remember staring down at my sons as they sucked down their bottles, wondering how their lives might unfold. I imagined them as boys playing little league, as teenagers on their first dates, as young men heading off to college. I dreamed that they'd grow up to be best friends.

In those early months I'd strap the boys into our side-by-side double stroller and walk the short distance from our apartment to downtown Great Neck. People always stopped me to exclaim, "Aw, twins!" And I can't count the number of times I heard, "Double the trouble!" That always surprised me. Couldn't they see how delicious my sons were? How lucky I was? I'd smile and respond, "No, double the pleasure!"

Even though we had our share of colicky crying jags and sleepless nights, that first year was infused with joy. A sense of promise followed me everywhere, and I know I will always remember their infancy swathed in the idyllic glow of new love.

I was home with the boys for almost four months, and then we hired a nanny to take care of them when I returned to work. Barbara was a lovely woman originally from Jamaica, and she adored the boys. I was working in a large nonprofit agency, but my office was close enough for me to come home and feed the boys over lunch. Allan's real estate office was close by, as well, so he regularly checked in on them during the day, as did my parents, who lived in nearby East Meadow. We couldn't get enough of those babies.

When they could pull themselves up, they'd stand in their cribs and throw all their stuffed animals out onto the floor, erupting into giggles. They were the dickens, always getting into everything, climbing up on tables and in and out of cupboards. But they were so joyful about their mischief that it was hard not to laugh along with them.

They met all their developmental milestones—rolling over, sitting up, walking—early. And just before their first birthday, I was holding Jamie in the boys' room when he pointed at the huge stuffed bear hanging on the wall and said his first word: "bear!" I yelled to Allan, who was in the other room with Alie, and said, "Come here! Jamie just said his first word!"

We celebrated the boys' first birthday at my parents' house on June 16, 1991—Father's Day—amid blue and white balloons and *Happy Birthday* banners. I loved the fact that we could celebrate their birthday on Father's Day. It seemed that they were somehow blessed, sharing the day with Allan and my dad. Allan and I were very close to my parents, and I hoped that Alie and Jamie would grow up to be as close to Allan and me as we were to my mom and dad.

My parents adored Alie and Jamie. My sister Edie had two sons, Eric and Richard, who were 11 and 12 years old, and I know my parents had hoped Allan and I would have children, too. But when Allan was diagnosed with multiple sclerosis four years earlier and began to struggle with fatigue, muscle pain, and headaches, we weren't sure if we should—or could—have children. His first MRI showed a number of lesions on his brain where the myelin sheath around his nerves had been damaged. The doctors explained that prognosis varied from person to person and told him he might develop a relapsing/ remitting pattern or simply become progressively worse. Regardless, it would make life unpredictable.

That aspect of the disease—not knowing what lay ahead—alarmed us both. So when we found out I was pregnant—with twins no less!— we were terrified. But that terror quickly turned to joy, and soon neither of us could imagine our lives without Alie and Jamie. We both embraced parenthood with the enthusiasm with which we tackled everything. Their first birthday was filled with friends and family and lots of laughter. The boys messily ate huge pieces of cake, they wrinkled and tore at the colorful wrapping paper on their presents, and they played Ring-Around-the-Rosie with my friends' children, laughing when they all fell down. And they were so attentive, running into our arms when we called their names.

The months following their birthday passed in a blur of activity: we watched the boys chase each other around our apartment in their walkers, we took them for long walks into town or to the park, and we visited friends and my parents and Edie and her family. We had developed a routine, and I was so grateful for the life we'd built. Allan was, for the most part, able to manage his MS symptoms with a medley of vitamins and lots of rest. He experienced a few flare-ups— severe headaches and debilitating fatigue—but luckily they were short-lived and he didn't allow them to dampen our joy. We were, quite simply, happy.

But by 16 months old, the boys' development seemed to have slowed down. Jamie could still say "bear," but that was it, and Alie didn't have any language at all.

"Shouldn't they be talking?" Allan would ask, and I'd feel a tug of worry.

"Do you think they're behind?"

I began watching other toddlers at the park and noticed that some could say a handful of words. Were the boys behind? At their 17-month checkup, I asked our pediatrician if they were on track, and he reassured me that they would talk in their own time. After all, they were twins and had been born five weeks early.

But it wasn't just their lack of speech that began to worry Allan and me; they seemed to have changed. They no longer ran to us when we called their names, they no longer made eye contact, and sometimes they seemed distressed for no reason at all. When I handed them a ball or the stacking musical rings they loved just a month earlier, they now didn't seem interested at all. Sometimes when we were eating dinner, Alie would begin to shriek and squirm in his highchair, scattering food everywhere. Nothing we did calmed him down. And at the park, Jamie would twirl and jump, happily absorbed in his own world. But if he got sand in his shoes, he would dissolve into a fit of crying.

But maybe all of that was normal? They were our only children. We had nothing against which to compare their behavior or development. So what did we know? Maybe that's how toddler boys acted. In retrospect, the signs were clear: they had stopped pointing to things they wanted, they no longer responded to us, and they had started to engage in repetitive behaviors—tapping, jumping, flapping. But even if I had known that this wasn't normal behavior I wouldn't have known what it meant.

Finally, when they were 21 months old, Allan and I decided we should see a specialist. "It can't hurt," Allan said, both of us craving reassurance that our sons were okay.

Our pediatrician agreed that maybe that would be a good idea, and he wrote down the name of a neurologist. I called her office immediately.

It was March, and the day of our appointment was sunny and cold. Dr. Bergtraum's office was only ten minutes away from our apartment, and as I drove there, the boys in their car seats, I was anxious, my stomach in knots. But I was also relieved to be getting an expert's opinion.

I pulled into the parking lot of the office building, slung my purse and the diaper bag over one shoulder, then unbuckled and picked up a boy in each of my arms. Allan and I had gotten used to tag teaming, but I usually took them to their doctor's appointments on my own. There was no sense in both of us taking time off work.

I pushed open the door to Dr. Bergtraum's office and was met by a smiling receptionist. I checked in and then tried to entertain Alie and Jamie with a book while we waited. But neither of them would stay seated, instead running back and forth and jumping, jumping, jumping. Finally I lured them over to a train track that was set up in the corner, but instead of moving the cars back and forth on tracks, they banged them together again and again. The receptionist smiled empathetically. I felt my stomach clench. *What is going on with my sons?*

Once we were called into Dr. Bergtraum's office, I situated the boys on the floor with toys and settled myself in the chair opposite her desk. I had dressed the boys in different colored shirts and pants to be sure the doctor could tell them apart, but I needn't have worried. They were each fixated on their own thing. Within seconds, Jamie was up, heading for her file cabinet, opening and closing a drawer: *rattle, slam. Rattle, slam.* Alie crawled under her desk and then was out again, in and out, moving, always moving. Neither one of them responded to the doctor when she said their names. *Is this normal?* I wondered. Then, *No, they're fine. They're just active boys.*

Dr. Bergtraum seemed immune to the chaos the boys were causing around her. She straightened her suit coat and smiled, asking me quietly about my pregnancy, the birth. I answered her, explaining that the twin pregnancy had been a surprise but that I hadn't had any complications. She asked about the boys' attention spans, and I motioned toward them. "They fixate on things like this, but it's hard to get them to stay focused on a book or a game. They're always moving," I said, my voice suddenly shaky, almost a whisper. There was something about the questions, her calm voice, the way that she looked at the boys that unnerved me. Something must be wrong.

Dr. Bergtraum nodded her head and took notes as I spoke. Then she leaned back in her chair and watched the boys silently for two minutes, four, six. I watched her watch them and thought, *That's it? Aren't you going to say anything else?*

Finally she said evenly, "The boys have a language delay with autistic characteristics."

The gray walls of her office slanted, closing in on me. My ears buzzed. My chest seemed to compress, pressing the air from my lungs. I didn't even know what autistic meant; it was 1992, and people weren't talking about autism. But I knew it couldn't be good. Finally I said, "What's autistic?"

What did she say then? Something about a neurological disorder, about brain development. But it was hard for me to focus, to decipher her words. I wanted to pick up the boys and flee. As if I could outrun the diagnosis, protect us from what lay ahead.

Dr. Bergtraum probably delivered this kind of news all the time, and I wondered how she could stand it. She pursed her lips as she wrote down the diagnosis for me—*language delay with autistic characteristics*. She also listed a few agencies to contact and said the boys would need early intervention. I knew, in that moment, that my life was about to change forever.

In the parking lot I took deep breaths, letting the cold sting my lungs as I buckled the boys into their car seats. *Breathe. Everything is going to be fine.* But when I slid into the driver's seat, my hands were trembling. Alie began thrashing in his car seat, so I turned the key in the ignition. *I can't start crying now. I just have to get home. I just need to get my boys home.*

When we got to our apartment building I rushed to the elevator with a boy clutched in each arm, hoping I wouldn't see any of our neighbors, especially my friend Caren, who also lived there. Caren and I had been friends as kids but had lost touch until Allan and I moved into the apartment building. She had two sons, who were older than Alie and Jamie, and she'd given us tons of hand-me-down clothes for the boys. We now chatted regularly, and if she saw me, she'd know something was wrong. And what would I say? How could I describe the way my life had just changed when I didn't even understand it?

Thankfully, we didn't run into anyone. Back in the apartment, I strapped Alie and Jamie into their walkers and piled toys on their trays, hoping to keep them entertained. Then I dialed Allan's work number. For the last ten years Allan had been selling real estate on Long Island, and I hoped he'd be at his desk rather than out showing property. I held my breath until he picked up the phone.

"Hello," he said.

"You have to come home now." Suddenly, I was crying and I couldn't stop.

"Are the boys okay?" he asked.

"Yes," I said, but that was all I could manage.

"I'm on my way." I didn't ordinarily break down like that, so he knew it was bad.

Then I collapsed on the kitchen floor and cried, my head in my hands. How could this be happening? They're just babies, so innocent.

I started to pray: *please, please, God, help me. Please help my babies.* Maybe the doctor was wrong. Maybe they're fine. From the other room, I could hear the banging of toys on the boys' walker trays. Bang. Bang. Bang.

I glanced up at a photograph of Alie and Jamie that was propped on the dining room shelf. In it, they wore identical red and white outfits while lying on a blanket facing each other, propped on their elbows. A mirror image. They were smiling. They were looking into each other's eyes. Why weren't they doing that now? What went wrong?

Suddenly, I needed to hear my parents' voices. They had always been my biggest supporters. I picked up the phone again and dialed their number.

"Hello, hello, hello!" Dad answered, full of exuberance, as always.

Everything came rushing out: the questions Dr. Bergtraum asked, the way she watched the boys, the diagnosis. Dad asked what was next and I told him about the list of specialists.

"Robyn, listen to me. I promise you we will get through this," he said resolutely.

And in that moment I knew that somehow we would. Dad was my rock, and if he said we'd get through it, we would. He had always been unflappable, a problem solver, and I knew he would be able to help us navigate this nightmare.

Then my mom was on the phone. "Oh Rob," she said. Her voice caught. Mom and I were very close, and I knew she could feel my pain. I started to cry again. But Mom said, "It's going to be okay. We're here for you. Whatever you need, whatever the boys need. It's going to be okay." Mom had been a special education teacher in Long Island public schools for over 15 years, so even though she surely understood the gravity of the diagnosis and what it meant for us, she didn't let on.

"We're coming right over," she said.

"Thank you," I managed.

After I said good-bye to my mom, I stared at the phone in my hand and then at the sheet of paper Dr. Bergtraum had given me. I could hear the wheels of the boys' walkers clicking in the living room. Then they both began to whine loudly. Everything that had been important to me before—home, work, my new car, shopping for clothes for the boys—seemed to fall away. All that mattered now was my sons, my angels. And their future. I took a deep breath. *I have to be strong*, I thought. *They will be okay. They have to be okay.* So I dialed the first number and, with a halting voice, requested an appointment for an evaluation.

When I hung up, the boys were crying, and I knew they were done with their walkers. I stood up, and, even though I felt hopeless and terrified by the way our lives seemed to be unraveling, and even though I didn't want to believe that they were autistic—whatever that was—I loved my boys with all my heart, and I'd do anything for them. Whatever this was, I'd fix it.

In the living room, I pulled them from the confines of their walkers and hugged their squirming bodies to my chest. I sat down with them on the couch and kissed their soft faces and ran my fingers through their fine, dark curls. They tried to wiggle free, but I held them more tightly. Over and over again I said, *I love you. Mommy loves you. I love you so much.*

2

WHEN ALLAN ARRIVED HOME a few minutes later, he burst through the door, his brow furrowed. "What did the doctor say?"

I put the boys back into their walkers, and they resumed their frenetic racing and banging. I motioned to Allan to follow me, and in the kitchen I handed him the piece of paper from Dr. Bergtraum. The color drained from his face, and when he looked up, his blue eyes were full of fear.

"What do we do now?" he asked. But before I could answer he said, "What the hell! How are we going to manage?" I knew Allan was scared. If having MS was like living with a time bomb, stress was the match that ignited it. How would we navigate his MS *and* two sons with a *language delay with autistic characteristics?* Allan threw his arms out to his sides. "Rob, the way my MS symptoms are flaring up I could be headed for a nursing home, and you could be dealing with this on your own."

I knew that, of course. Still, I felt a spark of anger. Our world—the idyllic world we had inhabited since the boys were born—had been shattered, and I needed him to comfort me. Instead I was going to have to comfort *him.* I was scared, too—terrified—but instead of letting that fear paralyze me, it propelled me into action. So I squashed my anger with resolve. I hugged him tightly and then I looked into his tear-rimmed eyes. "We will do everything humanly possible for Alie and Jamie, and we will do it starting *now.*" Determination seemed to coil through my core, holding me upright. "And I will handle it. I will handle everything."

"You can't do this on your own," he said, defeated.

"I can," I said. "And I will."

But when my parents showed up a half hour later, I knew I would never have to deal with this new reality on my own. Dad folded me into a tight bear hug, and I let myself relax just a little, feeling safe, as I always did in his presence. Then my mom hugged me, her thin arms wrapping around my back. When she finally pulled away, she looked into my eyes, brushing the hair from my forehead. "It's going to be okay, Rob. The boys are going to be okay."

Her hazel eyes were filled with love as she squeezed my hand. I knew if she could somehow undo this diagnosis, she would. "I'm going to contact some of my colleagues and the director at Rosemary Kennedy."

I felt a pang of dread. Mom had worked with developmentally disabled kids for years. She had loved her work, called them "her" kids, rejoiced in every breakthrough, in each accomplishment, but the school depressed me—all those kids with such severe and sometimes dangerous behaviors. Whenever I visited her classroom, I was filled with sadness. And then Mom had been forced to retire early after one of her students—in the throes of a violent tantrum— kicked and punched her so hard that he dislocated two disks in her spine and she lost consciousness. The fact that my boys—my perfect boys—now needed that school's help made me feel nauseated. From the other room, we could hear Alie and Jamie scooting around, squealing.

Dad put one arm around me and one arm around Allan. "We're going to figure this out." Dad was the one, who, after Allan had been diagnosed with MS, convinced him to begin taking a medley of vitamins and wean himself from the medications he had been prescribed, the side effects of which were almost worse than his MS symptoms. Dad was a huge believer in naturopathic medicine and spent countless hours researching the right combination of vitamins that might help Allan. Though Dad wasn't a doctor—he'd been an accountant for years—Allan trusted his judgment, and he was right to do so. Although Allan still had regular flare-ups, his symptoms weren't getting progressively worse as we feared they might.

That day, Dad looked pensive, the edges of his mouth turning down, and I knew he was sad. But I could tell he was already planning, calculating how he could take us under his wing and protect us.

———

The ground was shifting under our feet, but I was determined not to fall. When I returned to work I requested a meeting with the executive director. I wanted so badly to quit my job and focus all my attention on Alie and Jamie, but I knew quitting wasn't possible; we couldn't afford for me not to work, especially because if I lost my job, we'd lose our health coverage. But I was hoping for an extended leave of absence. I had been with the company for 14 years, working my way up to deputy director, a fact I hoped would be taken into consideration. Not to mention that we were a human services agency meant to help people in need.

This was before the Family and Medical Leave Act went into effect in 1993, so obtaining time off to care for a sick child or family member was dependent primarily on supervisor approval. My boss watched me intently from behind her desk, nodding sympathetically as I described the diagnosis and the next steps, so I was hopeful my request for a leave would be granted. But when I finished talking, she sighed loudly. "Well, this is a no-win situation."

I felt as if I had been slapped. She was talking about my life, my children. A "no-win situation"? But she agreed to let me take a couple of weeks off to get my head around the diagnosis, and then unpaid time off to attend therapy sessions and doctors' appointments when needed. I was grateful.

———

I was desperate to learn as much as possible about what my boys were facing. But this was before the Internet transformed access to information. It was before advocacy organizations like Autism Speaks even existed. So I went to the Great Neck Library, sat at a long wooden table, and flipped through a stack of psychology books and papers. One of the first things I read was a paper by Leo Kanner, the psychologist who first identified autism in 1943. But the more I read, the sicker I felt. Kanner claimed that a lack of parental warmth and attachment caused autism in children, specifically a "genuine lack of maternal warmth." I looked up around the library. The sun shone outside, filling the large room with bright light. A couple of teenagers sat in front of the card catalogue, giggling. An elderly woman walked by me and smiled, a stack of books in her arms. How could all of these people be here, living their normal lives when everything I thought I knew about my life and how it would unfold now meant nothing?

I glanced back to Kanner's paper, feeling light-headed. *Is this my fault? Did I somehow cause my sons' autism?* It didn't matter that I smothered Alie and Jamie in kisses every chance I got. It didn't matter that I modeled my parenting on the warmth and closeness of my own parents; I suddenly felt like a failure. I pushed the other documents to the center of the table and stood, needing to hold my sons in my arms.

When I arrived home, the boys were taking a nap. Mom and Dad, who were babysitting, sat together on the couch reading. I broke down as I told them about Kanner's claim.

Dad was furious. "Don't pay any attention to that garbage," he said. "That was debunked years ago. Both Kanner and Bettelheim with his 'refrigerator mother.'" He shook his head. "Ridiculous."

Oh my god. I hadn't even heard the term "refrigerator mother."

Mom stood up and pulled me into a hug. "Robyn, you know that's the farthest thing from the truth."

"You have to read this," Dad said, handing me a book. I glanced down at its cover: *Infantile Autism: The Syndrome and its Implications for a Neural Theory of Behavior* by Bernard Rimland. "I've already been in touch with him, and he's recommended other reading." Dad smiled gently.

Even though I knew they were right, that Kanner's theory couldn't possibly be true, I continued to weep. Mom handed me a tissue and hugged me again. Finally I took a deep breath and shook my head, trying to banish Kanner's words from my mind.

"Go check on them," she said and I nodded.

I turned the handle as quietly as I could and stepped into the boys' darkened room. They were both sound asleep on their tummies in their cribs, their little legs tucked up beneath them. As I watched their backs rising and falling, rising and falling, I felt my chest expand with love, and my own breathing slowed. "I love you so much. I love you so much," I whispered into the quiet room. Carefully, I bent over the edge of Jamie's crib and kissed him on the back of his head. Then I did the same with Alie. *You're perfect*, I thought. *You have to be okay.* Then I stepped into the center of the room, taking in the photo-lined walls and stuffed animals, the rocking chair where I spent hours holding first one of them, then the other. *How can this be? How can you have autism? I couldn't have caused this, could I? What will happen to you, my sweet boys?*

———

That night, after the boys were in bed, Allan and I sat together on our beige leather couch, a stack of papers between us. I started to cry again as I told him about Kanner's theory.

"That's bullshit, Rob, and you know it." He leaned forward and pushed his glasses onto his forehead. "I can't believe you're taking that seriously."

"I know," I said, shaking my head and wiping away the tears with the back of my hand. "It was just so hard to read."

Allan squeezed my thigh, then picked up one of the articles from the couch. But after staring at it for a moment, he put it down again. "What else did you find out?"

I pulled one of the articles from a stack my dad had given me a few days earlier. I flipped through it until I found the highlighted checklist of autistic characteristics. "Listen to this," I said, and read them aloud to Allan: no eye contact, no response to name or smiles, no back-and-forth gestures such as pointing and reaching, no words, repetitive behaviors, flapping of arms.

"Oh my God," Allan said. "That's Jamie and Alie. How could we not have known?"

"I know," I said, guilt sliding through me and settling in my stomach. What we thought were just minor delays were clearly signs of autism. We could see it clearly now. Would it have mattered if we'd caught it a couple of months earlier?

I leaned into Allan, resting my head on his chest, and he put his arm around me and squeezed me tightly. Allan and I had known each other—had been together—so long that we didn't need to talk. I was 15 and Allan was 18 when we started dating—a lifetime ago. That had been a different time: the mid-70s, the age of bellbottoms and discos. Allan had been tall and thin with long blond hair and a full beard. We met at a party, and I was immediately attracted to him. But the thing I loved most about him was his sense of humor; he could make me laugh until I cried. We spent hours together doing nothing but laughing.

Those days now felt like a distant memory, and I wondered if we'd ever laugh like that again.

Allan reached for my hand. I knew he wished he could do something to take away my pain, our pain, and he would have done anything possible to make that happen. I knew how helpless he was feeling. I felt the same way.

"We have to figure this out," he said quietly.

I nodded. "We will," I said, trying to sound more positive than I felt.

———

The next morning, a special education teacher and a psychologist came to our apartment to evaluate the boys. I invited them to sit in the living room where Alie and Jamie were flapping their hands, twirling, jumping, running.

The special education teacher, Janet, was in her mid-fifties. She looked as though she was heading to a business meeting in black slacks and a freshly pressed blouse. Her dark hair was cropped short, and though she smiled when we shook hands, it was a smile that didn't reach her eyes. The psychologist, on the other hand, cupped my hand in both of hers and smiled warmly. She was dressed casually in a long flowered skirt and a beige sweater. Her dark blonde hair was pulled back loosely in a hair clip. "I'm Elizabeth," she said softly, as if she could sense my fear, as if she knew that I was clinging to hope that they would tell me that Dr. Bergtraum was wrong, that the boys were perfectly normal.

But as I watched Janet and Elizabeth observing the boys, who were lost in their chaotic movement, I knew that hope was futile. Again I was stunned that I ever believed this behavior was normal.

Janet pulled a clipboard from her black briefcase and shuffled papers into a neat stack on her lap. "We just need to ask you a few questions, and then we'll work with Alex and Jamie," she said, pulling out a pen.

I put the boys into their walkers so I could focus, and Janet proceeded to ask one question after another, all reminiscent of the questions that Dr. Bergtraum had asked: Did I have any complications with my pregnancy? What was the boys' birth weight? Did I have anemia?

I watched as Janet jotted down my answers on her clipboard, the boys careening around the room in their walkers, slapping their hands against the plastic toys that encircled them. What does all this mean for my sons?

When Janet exhausted her questions, Elizabeth asked me to move Alex and Jamie from their walkers to the floor. "We're just going to try a few things with the boys," Elizabeth said, smiling again. I felt my body begin to tense as I watched both women sit on the floor in front of my sons.

Janet waved at Alie. "Alex," she said. "Alex, look at me."

Alie pushed himself to his feet and ran to the bookshelf, turned and ran in a circle, his gaze unfocused. *What is going on in there, Alie?* I silently willed him to look at her.

She turned her attention to Jamie, who was up, as well, now jumping, jumping, jumping, his arms twirling in large circles. "Jamie, look at me. Jamie."

No response.

Janet then pulled a plastic bottle of bubbles from her bag. Alie was now facedown on the carpet on his stomach. Just lying there, licking the carpet. Janet blew bubbles near his face. I wanted to pull him into my lap. I reached out to help him up, but Elizabeth put out her arm. "No," she said gently, shaking her head.

I cringed, hating to leave him like that.

Finally Alie looked up at the bubbles and Janet said, "Good looking at the bubbles, Alie!" Her voice was high, too cheerful, and I felt a moment of relief. See, he's going to be fine. He can look at bubbles!

When Jamie stopped jumping long enough to look at the bubbles, she praised him, as well: "Very nice Jamie looking at the bubbles!"

She tried to get them to follow the bubbles and then say "Pop!" when the bubbles popped. But the boys had reverted to their jumping and licking.

Finally Janet twisted the cap back on the bottle and slid it into her bag as she sat back on the couch. "That they responded at all is a good sign," she said.

Somehow hope and despair wove together in my chest. Hope because a "good sign" is just what it sounds like. Despair because I was supposed to be reassured that, after dozens of attempts, my sons finally noticed the bubbles that floated and dipped in the air around them, something that would be a source of delight for a normal toddler.

"So what do you think?" I asked. "What does this all mean for my sons?"

The two women exchanged a glance, and I held my breath. I knew they didn't want to confirm what we all already knew.

Elizabeth brushed a few wisps of hair from her face. "We can't say exactly. Every child is different." She paused. "But we agree with Dr. Bergtraum's diagnosis." Her voice was soft, almost apologetic. "Language delay with autistic characteristics."

———

That night, I lay in bed unable to sleep, my mind racing. What next? Elizabeth and Janet left me with pamphlets and other numbers to call. I was to set the boys up with weekly speech therapy, occupational therapy, and special education. How would we coordinate it all?

Allan was snoring softly next me, and I wondered, irritated, how he could sleep. How could he go to work and come home and continue to eat and sleep when our sons' future was at stake? I felt utterly alone, and turned toward my bedside table, where there was a photo of the boys. It was taken a few weeks after their first birthday. They were sitting side-by-side in the stroller, both drinking juice from bottles, their blue onesies each proclaiming "BOY!" I smiled at the words on Alie's visor—Teething is the Pits—but then felt my throat tighten. Both boys were looking directly at me, smiling as they sipped their juice. They knew me. They responded. They were fine.

Now they no longer responded when we called their names. They seemed lost in their own worlds. How could I get them back? I started to cry, my body shaking with quiet sobs. "Please God," I whispered into the room. "Please help me. Please cure my sons. Please give me the strength to help them recover. Please."

3

OUR LIVES FELL INTO A KIND of rhythm after that first assessment—if it's possible to find rhythm in the chaos of navigating work and research and the boys' many therapy appointments; if it's possible that one can discover an unexpected cadence by stringing together the notes of confusion and heartbreak with dogged determination.

But underneath everything we were doing for the boys was the fear that it wasn't enough, that we were too late. Again and again we heard—from the therapists, in the articles that my dad continued to bring over—that early intervention was the key to success. So intervene we did. Within a week of the assessment, the boys had twice-weekly appointments with occupational therapists, speech therapists, and special education teachers. Their nanny, Barbara, still cared for them most weekdays, but I rushed home from work to relieve her for each appointment. I wanted to be there, soaking up as much knowledge as I could. I wanted to take part in their treatment. But I found it difficult not to help the boys, not to jump in and try to engage them, which of course defeated the purpose of the therapy.

Finally one of the therapists told me gently that my presence was distracting. "Oh," I said. "Of course." From then on during their multiple sessions a week, I sat on the floor in the hallway around the corner from the living room, trying to listen to exactly what they were saying: the repeated questions, the positive reinforcement when one of the boys made eye contact or stopped spinning through the room.

But some days they seemed to spend the whole hour screaming and crying, and I'd hold my head in my hands and cry, as well. Those were the days I wondered how they would ever make progress.

———

When the boys were two years old, we enrolled them in the Variety Child Learning Center, which provided early intervention and special education preschool services. It was about 20 minutes away in Syosset, Long Island. Dr. Bergtraum had mentioned it the day she diagnosed the boys, but it took me a few months to even contemplate sending them off to preschool on one of those mini buses. The program was only two hours a day, though, and Allan and I decided that the more exposure they had to services, the better. I was still nervous about sending the boys on the bus alone, so I arranged to have Barbara ride with them there and back and help out in the office while the boys were in class.

I felt heartsick that first day. Allan and Barbara and I stood outside our apartment with the boys strapped into their stroller, which Allan pushed back and forth as we waited for the bus to arrive. Barbara squeezed my hands, which were shaking. "They're going to be okay," she said, her Jamaican accent thick, somehow reassuring. "I'll be with them."

"I know," I said, feeling a wave of gratitude, gratitude for the fact we had a place like Variety to send Alie and Jamie, gratitude for Barbara, for her warmth and love for the boys. I knew there were other parents dealing with autism who didn't have the resources we had, or didn't know how to get connected to those resources.

Still, I hated sending them to Variety on the bus that day. It was as if, by sending them to a school for kids with developmental disabilities, I was giving up, giving in to their autism, admitting that they needed more intensive services than we could provide at home. I thought of my cousin Billy, who had severe cerebral palsy and cognitive disabilities.

As a little girl I had been scared of him, scared of the ways he was different, the jutting angle of his jaw, the twisted claws of his hands. But he always had a huge smile on his face, and my aunt Frances was always smiling, as well. As a child I wondered how my aunt could be so happy with such a disabled son. He spent his days in a program for people with disabilities, and now I was terrified that Alie and Jamie would end up in a program like that, as well. I couldn't bear it. And I couldn't imagine actually smiling through it. What about college and girlfriends, marriages and families of their own someday?

———

At Variety the boys did activities typical to preschoolers: coloring with crayons, making collages with construction paper and too much glue, playing with Play-Doh. But they needed constant supervision to stay focused. I had learned that both boys had stereotypy, the persistent repetition of behaviors that serve no functional purpose but provide sensory stimulation, which often occurs with autism. Jamie would suddenly jump up from the table and lunge toward the window or begin his obsessive jumping. Alie was easily distracted and would soon be lost in a streak of sunlight on the floor. He was mesmerized by light and shadows, and it was difficult to call him back. Or he would begin tapping his fingers on the table or stomping his foot, caught in a loop of repetitive movement. I stopped by the preschool almost daily and peeked through the window, watching with a sinking heart as the teachers tried to redirect them again and again and again.

The afternoons were filled with therapy appointments in our living room. The occupational therapist sat cross-legged on the floor, trying to get the boys to roll a ball back and forth with her, to make eye contact, to respond to their names. Sometimes they would roll the ball, sometimes they would make eye contact, but not consistently. Often they would fixate on the shag of carpet or the sound of a toy car banging against a book. The speech therapist explained to me that she was working on developing their receptive language when she would ask the boys to show her the book or toy they were holding. She was trying to gauge their understanding of language. Alie and Jamie rarely did as she asked. They didn't understand. Sometimes she would pull a *Sesame Street* puppet or musical organ from her bag and ask which one they wanted. "Point to the toy you want." They would grab or vocalize, but never point. During these sessions, the progress was slow if noticeable at all, and it felt as if we were stuck in quicksand, slowly sinking despite all our efforts.

In the evenings, after Allan and I put the boys to sleep, we'd sit together on the couch and I'd summarize the boys' therapy sessions, how things were going, but I tried to keep it simple and I often omitted bad news—their lack of progress, how concerning it was that they wouldn't eat anything besides apples and grapes and Goldfish. I hated to overwhelm Allan because he was in the midst of a flare-up and wasn't sleeping well due to muscle pain. And he was so busy. In addition to his real estate business, he also owned a small car sales and repair business. He was already burning the candle at both ends. The last thing I wanted to do was make him more stressed out. And I thought if I could stay positive, keep pushing forward, maybe it would all work out.

———

I could feel myself pulling away from the larger world. I wasn't interested in talking to anyone about the boys' diagnosis unless they were involved in their care or also had children with autism. And frankly, I didn't have the time. I needed to keep learning, keep surrounding myself with people and resources that could help us. My girlfriends were still there and we'd talk on the phone occasionally, but there was a growing distance between us. Maybe I was resentful, maybe I was exhausted, maybe both. I just knew that I could no longer invest the same amount of energy in my previous friendships.

I ran into my neighbor Caren one day as I was on the way to the park with the boys. I hadn't seen her for months, even though she'd dropped off a bag of clothes at our door a few weeks earlier. Had I even thanked her?

Her sons were four and five years old, and she held each of them by the hand as they walked toward us across the parking lot. I could feel my body tense.

"Robyn!" she said, smiling. "I haven't seen you for so long. How are you? How are the boys?"

I stopped the stroller on the sidewalk in front of her. "Oh, you know," I said, trying to keep my voice light. "We've just been so busy."

Caren brushed the bangs from her forehead, and her older son, Justin, leaned into her side. "You're getting so big!" I said, glancing from Justin and Andrew. Both boys smiled up at me, and I felt that now-familiar wave of jealousy. They understood me. They responded with smiles. They stood quietly next to their mom.

Just then Alie vocalized loudly and began pulling at the straps of the stroller. *No,* I thought. *Not now.* Caren looked down at Alie and her brow furrowed in concern. Both of her sons stared openly at him. I pushed the stroller back and forth with my foot, but Alie's cries only grew louder. I grabbed the small container of Goldfish crackers from under the stroller and handed a few to Alie. "It's okay, Alie. Alie, it's okay. Here's some Goldfish. You love Goldfish." Alie's face was contorted in frustration, and he batted my hand away.

"I guess they're ready for their walk," Caren said sympathetically. She leaned toward Alie. "Are you ready to go?"

I took a breath, grateful that she was giving me an out. They're just tired. They're ready to go. But I knew I'd have to tell her eventually, so I might as well do it now. I slipped a Goldfish into Alie's mouth, and he stopped thrashing. I put a few more in his lap and a few in Jamie's lap and stood up.

"Actually," I said, "the boys have been diagnosed with autism." I could feel the rock of dread settle in my stomach again. It was as if each time I said those words aloud, each time I broke the news to someone else, the boys' diagnosis became more real.

"Oh Robyn," she said, "I'm so sorry."

I don't know what most people thought when they heard "autism." Some people may have thought of Dustin Hoffman playing Raymond Babbitt in *Rain Man*. I had already learned how inaccurate that portrayal was; Babbitt was extremely high functioning while most people with autism weren't savants. And for some reason I hated that people might picture Raymond Babbitt as soon as I mentioned that Alie and Jamie had autism.

Caren reached out and squeezed my arm. "What can I do to help? I'm happy to do whatever I can."

She couldn't help me, of course. She couldn't help the boys. But I appreciated her warmth anyway. I could feel a sting behind my eyes and I shook my head slightly. I would not cry. Instead I smiled. "We're doing therapy every week and they're doing well. And they're going to preschool every morning. So, things are okay right now."

Caren nodded, her boys standing patiently at her sides. "Well let me know if I can do anything. I'm just down the hall, and I'd be happy to watch them if you need a break."

"Okay," I said, though I knew I'd never ask her to do that. Alie and Jamie were, quite simply, too much work. They were always moving, always screeching, always banging, always flapping. I, too, became frustrated with them, unable to decipher what they needed or wanted. I certainly wasn't going to ask someone with no experience with autism to take care of them. It would never work. Besides, I already felt guilty that I was away from them at work almost all day.

———

My dad was in full-blown research mode, each week dropping by with articles on treatments and therapies that showed promise. He began almost every phone conversation with, "So I was doing a little research...." He tracked down specialists across the country, and either he or I would call them, asking for referrals to anyone on the East Coast they thought might be able to help us. I wrote letters to autism experts in England. One consultant I hired insisted we focus on motor imitation, on how the boys formed vowels with their mouths. We spent weeks helping them move their mouths into an O position, with no sound coming out. He said that this was the first step to developing language, and it was necessary to spend an extended period of time on it. I wanted to believe this would help, but something didn't seem right about it. After weeks, I wanted to know when we could actually work on sounds, but he said that the boys weren't ready yet. I began to feel that he was stringing us along for the money. Not to mention that he was always checking his watch. One day I was in the middle of asking a question when he interrupted me to say that our time was up and that we'd finish our conversation the following week. But I was done. I needed direction, but direction backed by proven success, direction provided by someone who actually seemed to care about my sons.

That's when we began to hear more about ABA: applied behavior analysis. My dad came over one evening with a paper on ABA and handed it to me. "This is it," he said, smiling his wide smile. "This is promising."

The paper was by Dr. O. Ivar Lovaas, who had been doing research at UCLA on the use of behavior modification and ABA with children with autism. Typical children learn from their environment: when their parents smile at or praise them, they understand that they've done something good. Children with autism don't make that connection. Lovaas' research, instead of focusing on the treatment of autism, focused on teaching children with autism how to learn.

In 1986, Dr. O. Ivar Lovaas presented this paper at a conference in King of Prussia, Pennsylvania, about his research using one-on-one intensive (40–50 hours per week) ABA with young children with autism. The results were unprecedented: almost half the children in his study lost their diagnosis. They recovered from autism. At the time, the normal ratio of staff to children in early childhood classrooms was one staff person for every two to three children, and no one knew how a one-to-one ratio would ever be possible. It would be too expensive. The answer was parents and home-based ABA programs *run* by parents. Over the next few years, it would be parents who pushed for one-on-one intensive ABA. It would be parents who got the government agencies to see what their children were capable of, who demanded that their children receive the appropriate resources and interventions. It would be parents who reclaimed their children.

But I didn't realize that at the time. I was excited by what I was learning about ABA and its success rate, but I didn't know what it might mean for the boys until I read Catherine Maurice's memoir *Let Me Hear Your Voice*, about her journey navigating the world of autism and ABA therapy with two of her three children. It was published in 1993, when Alie and Jamie were three years old, and I devoured the book in a day and a half, mesmerized, unable to put it down. I saw Alie and Jamie in the descriptions of Maurice's daughter and son. I saw myself in Maurice's grief and determination. And, page by page, as I watched her children slowly recover from the disorder that had claimed Alie and Jamie, I felt hope rise like a balloon in my chest. With intensive ABA therapy—50 hours a week in their home—Maurice's children were cured. Both of them, cured.

Her book was a road map to recovery, and it made me more determined than ever. If she could do it, I could do it. I could cure my sons. As I read, I highlighted excerpts and wrote down the names of every doctor and therapist mentioned in the book. As soon as I finished reading, I began looking up contact information and making phone calls. I just needed the right person to guide me, to help me recover my sons.

4

THE LIVING ROOM IN OUR apartment had been transformed into a play room/therapy room. It was loud and chaotic. The boys often set each other off: if Alie was whining and began to screech or throw things, Jamie would start whining too and do the same. Then the two of them would be tantruming in tandem, banging toys and thrashing and kicking on the floor. I tried to be patient, to remind myself that this was their autism, that they couldn't help it—but the noise and the constant motion, and not always knowing what would set them off, was wearying. They were constantly taking toys from each other, which could spark a tantrum, as well, so we had to have duplicates of all their favorite toys. There were also two swings, two jumpers, and two walkers. Almost every afternoon, there was also a therapist (or two) camped out on the floor, working with the boys in the cramped space.

We clearly needed more room for the boys, but we also needed more room for Allan. Due to his MS, he suffered from extreme fatigue. By four o'clock each day, his eyes became red and glassy, all the energy from the morning drained away. He was capable of working the long hours required of him as a real estate broker and small business owner as long as he could lie down and rest every afternoon. But between the coming and going of therapists and Alie's and Jamie's inability to modulate their volume, it was difficult for him to get the sleep he needed to keep from exacerbating his MS. We needed more space. We needed a house.

We wanted to stay in Great Neck, but most of the homes in town were above our price range. Allan began keeping a close eye on new listings and we toured one old house after another, but most of them needed too much work. We did this for weeks until finally we found one that was perfect. It needed work, as well—the second floor wasn't finished—but it had a large living room with big windows, wide mahogany paneling, and built-in bookcases. The floor was covered in wide yellow pine planks. It had "old world" appeal—traditional and warm. There were also two bedrooms and a den on the first floor, and there was a shaded backyard where we could play with the boys.

After we closed on the house, we spent weeks peeling off wallpaper, tearing up carpet, stripping and restaining floors, retiling the kitchen, and painting. My parents came to babysit after we had put the boys to bed, and Allan would head over to the house to work into the night. It was exhausting but also invigorating. The house represented a new beginning for our family, a place we could all thrive. It filled me with optimism. I even hoped that Allan and I might carve out the space we needed to nurture our relationship, which, since the boys were diagnosed, had became strained. I couldn't understand how he could turn off his brain and watch the news or movies at night. He begged me to relax, insisted we needed to talk about something other than autism. But it was difficult for me to flip that switch. I couldn't stop the scroll of worries from unfurling in my head, not for a conversation and certainly not for long enough to make love to my husband.

———

Preparing for the move and readying the house slowed down my search for the right consultants for Alie and Jamie, but I was still attempting to contact the professionals from Maurice's book, following the trail of recommendations. A conversation with a therapist in Florida led me to an ABA specialist in New Jersey, which led me to Joanne

Gerenser, a speech pathologist at Staten Island's Eden II School for Autistic Children. I was excited to learn that there was a specialized school exclusively for children with autism so close by, and I was hopeful I would find the right person there to help us, but after our experience with less-than-stellar consultants, I was wary.

But then Joanne's name came up again when I spoke on the phone with Angela, another autism mom on Long Island. There was a tight network of autism parents on Long Island, and though I hadn't met many of them in person, I always felt relieved to connect over the phone. They understood what we were going through. We shared information and helped and learned from one another. Angela told me she had been consulting with Joanne about her son's severe autism, and she was really impressed. I had to at least talk to her, Angela said, and I agreed.

It only took a few minutes on the phone with Joanne for any doubts I may have had to vanish. She began to ask me questions about the boys, and when I told her that they were identical twins, I could feel her excitement. Maybe I *had* found the right person.

She explained that the work they were doing at Eden was based on scientific research, and then she described the impact that ABA was having on the kids there. "There's a little boy who, when he started here, couldn't sit still and focus on a simple task for more than two seconds without thrashing around and biting himself. Now he can focus on a task for 45 seconds." She laughed slightly. "It's so exciting to see that kind of progress." Joanne's voice exuded warm confidence.

I couldn't help feel excited, too. "I read a book," I said, "in which the author's children were cured of autism." I was hoping she'd say this was possible for the boys, too.

"Oh great!" she said. "You've already read *Let Me Hear Your Voice.*"

"Do you think that's possible for my sons?"

I held my breath as I waited for her answer.

"We've learned so much in the last 20 years," she said. "And Lovaas really helped revolutionize how we teach children with autism. The little boy I told you about is just one example. I've seen so many kids make amazing progress with ABA. But we need to get started right away."

I could feel my heart pounding. "Tell me what to do," I said.

"That's what I like to hear," she said.

We set up a time for the following week for Joanne to come to our house and meet the boys. When she arrived, Alie was running from room to room, crazed, unstoppable. Jamie was sitting on the floor by my feet, his dark hair tousled, pushing his index finger into the floor until it bent back. "Jamie, no," I said, dismayed, taking his hand in my own. I looked at Joanne, worried that despite her calm and confidence on the phone she might take one look at the boys and back out the door. But she wasn't fazed. She smiled, her light eyes earnest. "Okay, let's get started."

She had told me that she would begin with the ABA program right away that day, but first I had a million questions: How many of the children at the school have recovered from autism? How long did it take for them to speak? Are there any other books I should read? What are the ways that Allan and I can help with their recovery?

She patiently answered each of my questions, and I knew I was right to trust her. She seemed to know autism inside and out. Finally she said, "Let's take these little guys upstairs."

Allan had converted the unfinished upstairs of our house into a mini-school—two classrooms—so that when the therapists came to work with the boys they each had a separate space with small tables and toys.

I carried Jamie and Joanne carried Alie up the steps as they tried to wiggle free. When we got upstairs, Joanne said it would be best if she worked with the boys alone, and I nodded, though my heart sank. I wanted to see everything she did with them so I could replicate it.

But by this point I was accustomed to listening through doors so I sat down on the floor in the hallway outside the room, my ear against the wall. Both boys were crying. I heard Joanne giving them directions: "Alie, sit down." More crying. Then, softly, "No, Alie, sit down." Her voice was firm but gentle. Then again, "No, Alie, sit down." And finally, an exuberant "Yay!"

Then I heard Joanne address Jamie: "Jamie, quiet feet." A pause. "No, Jamie, quiet feet." Soft, but firm. "No, Jamie, quiet feet. Yay!" I would learn that this was classic discrete trial training: No. No. Yay!

There was more crying and screeching, but there was also Joanne's calm voice. And then suddenly it was silent. *What was going on in there? How did she get them to be so quiet?*

When Joanne opened the door a few minutes later, I couldn't believe it when I saw Alie and Jamie both sitting down on their red Fisher Price plastic chairs. I was ecstatic. I thought, *Whatever you just did, I need to learn it.* I almost cried from relief. "Can you show me how to do that?"

"Absolutely," she said.

"How many hours a day will they need this?"

Joanne tilted her head and just looked at me for a few seconds before she said, "Robyn, they need this every day, 24 hours a day."

I must have looked startled because she said again, "This is how it's going to be. Do you understand?"

Even though I had read Maurice's book and I understood that ABA therapy was intense, I somehow hadn't grasped the magnitude of what we were undertaking.

Joanne smiled. "We'll set up a program to cover at least 40 hours of ABA a week."

I had no idea how to do that, but I said, "Of course. Whatever you say."

Before she left, she handed me a list of materials we would need for the classrooms—two of everything.

I nodded. "Allan was planning on putting observation windows in the doors, as well. Would that be helpful?"

"Yes!" Joanne said. "I like the way you're thinking. But we need to move fast. Every moment of every day is a learning opportunity. They're already three and a half, and their brains are developing quickly."

I nodded, a lump in my throat.

"Hire a staff," she said. Then, "We're going to do this!"

"Hire a staff?" I had no idea how to hire a staff, much less pay them. How were we going to manage?

"Put an ad in the paper. They don't need to be autism experts. They just need to want to learn and they need to be kind and gentle." She paused. "And determined."

"Okay," I said and nodded, my mind already at work.

Years later, I'd understand the significance of this moment—our turning point. For us, ABA was the lifeline for Alie and Jamie. Without it, the boys might have wandered off and drowned or gotten hit by a car. And later, because of their self-injurious behaviors, they might have put their arms through a window or given themselves concussions by banging their heads on the wall. It makes me panicky to even think about it, but I know that without ABA my sons might have died. They certainly wouldn't have been able to live at home with us. And they definitely wouldn't have become runners.

———

That night, Allan and I sat together at the dining room table, our monthly budget spread before us.

"How are we going to make this work?" he asked, his chin resting on his cupped hand. He shook his head.

I took a sip of my wine, my mind tired as I contemplated juggling it all. Joanne said we needed no fewer than eight therapists. Eight! "We just have to make it happen."

Allan nodded, and we spent the next several hours looking at our income and expenses. We had our salaries and savings, of course, and certainly my parents would help. But even if my parents made a generous contribution, which I knew they would, we still wouldn't have enough money to cover the program, and who knew how long we were going to have to do it.

But both Allan and I knew in our hearts that ABA was the answer for Alie and Jamie, so we took the next step on faith: we would find the staff and hire them provisionally. Then we would figure out how to fund the gap in order to make it happen.

I researched other early intervention programs in the area and heard about the New York State Office for Mental Retardation and Developmental Disabilities (now known as the Office for People with Developmental Disabilities). I learned that through New York State's Medicaid Waiver they were providing funding for home programs in addition to center-based programs, but I wasn't sure how we could access this funding.

I couldn't believe it when several days later a woman from the Long Island Developmental Disabilities State Office called. She had received information about the boys and asked if she could come for a visit and meet them. She and another woman came to our house and sat across from Allan and me in our living room, describing how New York State had funding available to help families like ours. As Allan and I held hands, I described Alie and Jamie's needs and talked about the proven success of ABA. They listened carefully, impressed, I think, that we were hiring a staff and planning a training with Joanne. And they said that because we had two sons with autism, the chances of us getting funding were fairly good.

When they left with a line about how they'd be in touch soon, I was hopeful, but still nervous. If they decided not to fund us, how would we manage?

Allan and I were flooded with relief when they called the following week to tell us they would help fund our program. It felt like a much-needed break, and we were grateful.

———

I placed an ad in the Pennysaver and in local college newspapers, and I pinned up notices around town, as well as in speech and psychology departments at C. W. Post College and Queens College: "AUTISM: PSYCHOLOGY, SPEECH, SPECIAL ED – Work P/T with twin boys with autism in my home program. Training provided in ABA (Applied Behavior Analysis). Join our team of professionals. Flexible days and hours."

My parents had joined GASAK (Grandparent Advocates Supporting Autistic Kids) and had become friendly with the founders, Robert and Thelma Krinsky, whose grandson had autism. So my dad also asked them for recommendations, and they referred us to Gina, who was one of their grandson's favorite therapists. She was trained in ABA, and it felt as though we'd won the lottery when she agreed to work for us.

Lisa, who had been working at the party store in town, came to us via my ad in the Pennysaver. She had no experience with kids with autism, but she was bubbly and warm, so we hired her. And Christine arrived via a flyer I had posted at a local college. She was studying to be a speech and language pathologist and was bright and enthusiastic. Within three weeks we had a staff of eight, most of whom had never worked with children, much less children with autism.

———

When our team was assembled, I took more time off work, and Joanne came back to lead a three-day training. We set up a video camera on a tripod in our living room and all gathered in a circle around Joanne. Allan took the boys over to my parents' house so we wouldn't be distracted. Joanne sat in the corner, sunlight streaming in the window around her, and I thought how perfect that was for her to be illuminated like that.

The first day she gave everyone a crash course in autism. She described it as a complex neurodevelopmental disorder characterized by "gross deficits in language development," "pervasive lack of responsiveness to other people," "peculiar speech patterns," and "restricted, repetitive, and stereotyped patterns of behavior." I nodded, jotting down notes, even though we were living with these symptoms day in, day out.

The second day she introduced ABA therapy and explained how, in order to learn, a child with autism needs everything broken down to the smallest step possible. We would use discrete trial training to break down skills into their most basic components, then reward positive performance with praise and reinforcers. Joanne explained that the boys each needed specific positive reinforcers—things they liked—with which they could be rewarded when they responded correctly to a question or instruction.

That was an easy one. Alie loved grapes, so a grape would be his reinforcer. For Jamie, a slice of apple. To help motivate them, Alie and Jamie would each have a token board with five Velcro pennies. They would get a penny after a correct response, and when all five pennies were on the board, they would get their reinforcer: a grape or slice of apple. One of our first programs would be the motor imitation program. Under that program would be different motor skills we would teach the boys to imitate, such as raising their hands, clapping, and standing up.

In order to move from one skill to the next—from, for example, "sit down" to "stand up"—Alie and Jamie would have to master the first skill. In order for a skill to be considered "mastered" they had to successfully execute it 90 percent of the time over three days with three different people. Joanne explained that if Jamie only raised his hands when I asked him to do it, it might be because I'd asked him to do it in a specific way, inadvertently prompting him. The behavior had to be generalized so that if anyone—anyone in any environment—asked him to put his hands up, he could do it.

Our job was to teach the boys how to learn. I was fascinated and filled with hope. I wrote a feverish stream of notes.

On the third day, Joanne demonstrated how to run discrete trials with the boys, and it worked. You could feel the excitement in the room.

Joanne explained that we would be starting with 30 discrete trial programs, including motor imitation, following verbal commands, one-step directions, receptive object identification, expressive object identification, receptive pictures, expressive pictures, eye contact, colors, numbers, oral motor imitation, and categories.

"And after those 30 programs?" I asked, thinking that at some point we would graduate from ABA and discrete trials.

"We just keep going," said Joanne, smiling. "We just keep building on each mastered skill."

We just keep going. "Okay," I said, nodding.

By the end of the last day of training, some of the therapists looked tired, their eyes beginning to droop, and I felt a spark of irritation. *Pay attention. This is going to save my sons!* Looking back, I know I wasn't easy to work for, especially in those early months of the home program. It was unfair and unrealistic to expect everyone to give as much as I was giving in order to make the program work. It was, I later realized, unfair to expect it even of myself.

5

AFTER WE LAUNCHED OUR HOME program, it was as if we existed in two worlds: the real world and the world of ABA. ABA took over our home—we ate, slept, and lived it. I became accustomed to the sing-song praise, the repetition, the reams of data sheets we used to record each of the skills we were teaching Jamie and Alie. I stayed up until midnight or 1:00 AM every night, transferring the data from the day—the plus signs and check marks and minus signs denoting whether or not the boys had mastered a skill—into graphs so we could track their progress. Each skill in each of our daily discreet trials had to be recorded before I went to sleep at night.

In the beginning, Allan would try to convince me to watch a movie or go to bed, but I never did—I had to make sure everything was ready for the next day—and eventually he stopped asking. When I finally slipped into bed, he was usually asleep.

I didn't see any other way for it to be. We were living in a bubble—an intensive ABA lab—and for the most part the boys seemed to be doing well. In the first few months of our home program, they learned how to imitate and follow simple directions and identify objects and pictures. They were rapidly acquiring skills.

Learning was easier for Jamie than Alie. When we tried to get Alie to identify things he liked—apples, books, music—he was completely inconsistent. If we asked him to point to the apple, he'd sometimes point to the apple, other times to the music player or the book.

He couldn't seem to grasp the concept. But when you're using ABA and a child isn't making progress in a given period of time, something isn't right about the way you're teaching the material. So our first challenge was to figure out *why* he wasn't getting it; our second challenge was to find a way around that "why."

Around this time, Ruth Donlin and Randy Horowitz joined our team. Ruth had a background in psychology and was working with children with developmental disabilities in a day treatment program. She slid seamlessly into our home program and within days picked up the ins and outs of ABA and our discrete trials. Randy was a special education teacher at the Rosemary Kennedy School. I met her the previous year when we had taken the boys there for an additional assessment, and she was calm and gentle—clearly devoted to the kids she taught. Joanne knew Randy and had convinced her to consult with us on curriculum.

Ruth figured out that when we asked Alie to identify objects, there was a pattern to his answers. He was pointing to the objects in the same order—left, center, right—regardless of which object we had asked him to identify and what object was in that position. Randy then suggested we pair a physical sign with the object. For "apple" we put a fist to our cheek, for "book" we opened our palms like a book, and for "music" we put our left arm out with palm facing up and stroked our inner left arm with our right hand. And it worked! By combining a motor skill (one part of the brain) with the receptive language (another part of the brain) he suddenly was able to learn! You could tell by his face that he understood that he "got" it. He smiled a genuine smile, a smile that reached his blue eyes. Then we threw him in the air and tickled him. "You did it, Alie! You did it! Yay!" Those were the kinds of breakthroughs that kept me going.

———

Because the boys were making steady progress, I sometimes forgot how far behind they were developmentally. But then I would see a mother and her four- or five-year-old walking down the street in Great Neck jabbering away—having a real conversation—and it would hit me hard, how much work we still had to do, how far behind the boys really were.

One of my least favorite places became the park. At the age of four Alie and Jamie loved the swings, the feel of air whooshing into their faces, and the slides, which they would go down over and over again. They mostly did well. Jamie loved to watch the other children play. Sometimes he would approach another child and jump up and down garbling happily, wanting, I think, to play, but not knowing how to make that happen. Because one of the characteristics of autism is impaired social interaction, I was thrilled whenever I saw him wanting to connect with another child. But the other children simply looked at Jamie quizzically or became frightened and retreated to their mothers. When that happened, I think Jamie sensed their confusion and fear, and that broke my heart. Sometimes I prompted him to say hi, but since Jamie didn't understand the nuances of social interaction, that's as far as it went. And if something agitated Alie or disrupted him during one of his obsessions—tapping his feet on each of the slide steps or rubbing his face on the chain of the swing—I had to try to redirect him before his anxiety transformed into a tantrum. "Tantrum" isn't even the right word for it. It was more like a tornado. He became frenzied, flying in circles, screeching. I knew he was trying to communicate, to tell me what was wrong, but he couldn't. Instead, he became a twirling mass of chaos—snapping his wrists, scratching his arms, biting his knuckles, throwing whatever was in his path. Most often his destruction was focused inward—he would only hurt himself—but if I tried to hold him, calm him down, he sometimes hit or bit me. Looking back, I realize I couldn't blame the parents and kids who would stop and stare, startled fear written on their faces. But back then, I *did* blame them because it hurt so much to watch Alie spin out of control, it hurt that I couldn't keep him safe, and it hurt that other parents could stand there flanked by their normally developing children. So I stared back, sometimes adding, "My sons have autism."

That would usually soften them. "I'm so sorry," they'd say, or sometimes just, "Oh." But they would still move away, shepherding their seemingly perfect sons and daughters to the other side of the play structure. When they didn't respond at all, I felt rage uncoil in my belly, and I glared, my hands on my hips. "Is there a problem?"

———

A major issue we were having with Alie was pica, an abnormal desire to eat non-food items. He would eat tiny pieces of puzzles and crayons. He'd pull threads from a shirt or pillow and work those around in his mouth. He'd dig his nails into the wall for paint chips and he even began chewing on his bedframe. If we saw him do it, we could remove the item from his mouth. We would stay with him until he fell asleep. But alone in his room in the middle of the night, how could I keep him from chewing on his bed?

The word "pica" is Latin for magpie. It's said that the magpie will eat anything and everything. But while Alie couldn't discriminate between items he *wasn't* supposed to eat, he and Jamie both were very discriminating where real food was concerned. Part of this had to do with their rigidity; everything had to be exactly the same every day. And their obsessiveness seemed to be gaining strength. Alie would stack the puzzle boxes on the shelf in the family room so that the front of all the boxes were flush and would fly into a rage if the boxes slipped out of alignment. Jamie would arrange his crayons in a perfect line, each crayon label face up and in the same direction.

This rigidity and obsessive behavior spilled into their diets. The only things they would eat were apples, grapes, Goldfish crackers, and french fries—clearly not a healthful diet. So we had to develop an eating program. Our first target was bread, so we would place the tiniest piece of bread—smaller than a pinky fingernail—on a plate. On another plate there would be a grape for Alie, a slice of apple for Jamie. We said, "Okay, if you eat the bread," pointing to it, "you can have a grape or apple." But with Alie, especially, it was as if we were poisoning him. For weeks he would scream and cry, thrashing his head back and forth, refusing to touch the bread. When he finally put it on his tongue, we would explode with positive reinforcement—*Yay!*—and throw him up in the air and give him his grape. We ran the program—five trials—every half hour, every day, which amounted to fifteen times a day. We took data on every trial, recording a + if the boys ate the bread independently, a − if they refused it, a +P if they ate it but only when prompted, and a -P if they refused it even when prompted.

Once they had mastered larger and larger pieces of bread, we worked on Wheat Thins, Ritz crackers, Life cereal, corn muffins, and bananas. Sometimes it only took a day to master and generalize a food, other times it took longer. Later we moved on to macaroni, plain cheese, waffles, chicken, green beans, turkey, pizza, peas, potatoes, and on and on. Progress was slow, but it was progress, and I was still convinced that we could cure the boys of autism, just as Catherine Maurice's kids were cured.

Allan and I agreed that we'd try other, experimental treatments, as well, as long as they were safe and seemed promising. One doctor was making waves in autism circles with the use of antivirals and antifungals to treat children with autism. He was based in California but would fly to New York and meet with families monthly at a hotel in Westchester to prescribe medications and track progress. I always felt a little uncomfortable meeting with him in a hotel and paying him cash for the medicine—it felt clandestine. So after a few months, when we didn't notice any improvement in the boys, we discontinued that treatment.

Then I heard about a study that was being done at Mt. Sinai Hospital. Research suggested that neurocognitive disorders such as autism had an immunological component, so in this study they were giving children with autism monthly IVs of immunoglobulin (IVIG). Ideally it was supposed to increase eye contact and social interactions, and decrease hyperactivity; irritability; lethargy; stereotypy; and echolalia, the repeating or echoing of what another person has just said, something Jamie did. It seemed safe, and Allan and I agreed that the potential benefits outweighed the side effects, which could include headaches, chills, fever, nausea, abdominal pain, and increased blood pressure.

The study at Mt. Sinai was particularly interested in twins, so I was able to get the boys into it. Once a month, I drove them into New York City for their infusions, which took an hour each time. The boys were cooperative as long as I let them watch *Sesame Street* and *Barney* videos as they were infused. We did this for six months. The boys didn't seem to have any adverse effects from it, and we thought we saw some improvement—less irritability and more consistent eye contact—but we had hoped for more.

I was determined to do everything I could for my sons, to search out a cure for their autism, but I also realized that I was desperate. I would have done anything at all if I thought it would have helped them. Later I'd learn that that kind of desperation isn't uncommon for parents of children with autism. Research shows that parents of children with Down syndrome and other disabilities often accept their children's diagnosis much more quickly than parents of children with autism. Maybe this has to do with the fact that so many children with autism seemed like happy typical kids for their first year, before they slipped away.

I understood why parents resisted an autism diagnosis. Because I saw my boys recede before my eyes, it seemed impossible that there wouldn't also be some miracle treatment that would return them to me. Also, part of me still felt I was somehow responsible for their autism, that somehow it was my fault. And in order to alleviate my guilt, to keep it from engulfing me, I kept pushing, kept searching for a cure. I filled each available moment of each day with whatever therapy or treatment might make a difference, might bring them back to us.

6

THE YEAR THAT THE BOYS were home-schooled full time was a difficult one for Allan and me. There was little time for the two of us, and we argued a lot, often about the boys' learning. I had immersed myself in ABA and attended every team meeting, as well as outside conferences and autism workshops—anything that might help me help Jamie and Alie. Allan was involved in their care as well, of course, but he was only peripherally involved in their schooling and rarely attended team meetings. So occasionally he would handle one of the boys' behaviors differently than the team had decided to address it, and I'd snap at him. Then he'd become angry with me, and soon we were yelling at each other.

Allan also wanted us to try to have a semblance of a normal life and go out with friends occasionally or have a date night once in a while. It was easy for him to compartmentalize, to put the boys and even his MS aside in order to enjoy himself. Partly, this was his personality—he'd always been social and had a wide network of friends—but because of his MS, he had also learned the importance of sometimes putting himself first. He knew when he needed a break, when he needed to refresh. I couldn't do that. I had tunnel vision—everything was about the boys. I was envious of his ability to disconnect; at the same time, it enraged me.

Sometimes I wish I could go back to those early years and do them differently—take the time to nurture our marriage, to nurture myself. But it would be years before I would learn how to slow down and take care of myself.

We both worried that our marriage wouldn't withstand the stress of autism. There were days when I thought it would be easier to just do it on my own. But I also couldn't imagine a life without Allan; we had been together for half of our lives. And on good days, days when the boys seemed happy, when there were no tantrums, when they were learning, *really* learning, Allan could still make me laugh. In those moments, the armor in which I'd encased myself after the boys' diagnosis cracked open and fell away, and I let joy momentarily bubble to the surface. Those moments were fleeting and far between, but somehow they were enough to keep Allan and me tenuously tethered together.

———

Our home program was working—the boys were learning—but it wasn't sustainable, financially or emotionally. It also didn't make sense to do the work we were doing in isolation when places like Eden II existed.

When the boys were four and a half, Joanne secured two spots for them at Eden II in Staten Island, and I was thrilled at the thought of them being in a place where there were so many autism and ABA experts on hand. But Allan disagreed. "We can't make them sit on a bus for over three hours every day. It's too far!" We argued about it for days, and finally I relented. It was true that unless they were carefully supervised on the bus, Alie might have a tantrum and hurt himself or eat something that could make him sick. Even Jamie, who would go along with just about anything, struggled with sitting still for long periods of time.

When I told Joanne that Allan and I had decided we couldn't accept the placements at Eden, she understood. What we needed was an Eden closer to home.

"You know, Robyn, there are other families here on Long Island in the same situation. They're searching for the right place with the right services for their kids."

"I want to meet them," I said.

Joanne put me in touch with three other families who were also struggling with placement. Joanne thought that if we were able to raise enough money to help pay for teachers, staff, and rent, the Board of Directors of Eden II might agree to open a satellite program on Long Island. At the time there was a moratorium on new school development in New York, so the only way we could lobby for a school specifically for children with autism was to open one under the auspices of an already-existing school, such as Eden II.

The first time Allan and I met the other parents was in a church basement in Bellmore, Long Island, 20 minutes from our house. The pastor of the church had a son with autism, so we were warmly welcomed. But we also felt at home because for the first time since the boys were diagnosed, Allan and I were surrounded by other parents who were grappling with the same issues.

There were four other parents there: Angela, Ellen, Sharon, and Olga, and they all had children with severe autism who were a year older than Alie and Jamie. Angela was the parent who had first raved to me about Joanne on the phone the year before, and I was happy to finally get to thank her in person for the recommendation. The other parents had also been working with Joanne, and they were already friends, brought together by autism. They were as desperate for a school like Eden II as we were.

It was a relief to not have to explain to other parents what it felt like to navigate the constant meltdowns, the loud screeching, the stereotypy, the sleepless nights, the sensitivities to noise. We had all been indoctrinated in the autism club, so we just nodded and commiserated when one of us described an epic tantrum or an emerging obsession. It was also energizing to be with a group of parents who were filled with the same fire that consumed me. Together we would create a place where all our children could learn.

We had weekly meetings in the church basement and decided to call the satellite school the Genesis School. One of the parents suggested Genesis because of its connection to the Bible and creation. It also seemed to tie in perfectly with Eden, which in Hebrew means "delight or enjoyment." We all agreed; we'd be starting something new, something hopeful.

So we christened our project Genesis, hired a lawyer to help us establish nonprofit status, and began raising money. We wrote letters, made phone calls, and begged friends and family for donations. It took us months, but we raised over $100,000, the amount that Joanne thought would convince the Eden II Board of Directors that a satellite school on Long Island was not only needed, but feasible.

Joanne, who had become the Executive Director of Eden II, helped us prepare a proposal and budget, which Angela and I took with us to the next board meeting. Over a dozen board members, some parents, some autism experts, and some community members were seated at an old rectangular wooden conference table. My heart pounded as we handed out our documents and took our seats at the head of the table. This felt like our one chance, and I was petrified. What if they didn't approve it? What if we had to go back to the drawing board? Who else would sponsor a school like this? We passed out copies of the budget, and I described how the money we had raised could augment the cost of the first year. I passed around pictures of Alie and Jamie and the other children in our group, describing each of their personalities, behaviors, and intense needs.

When I was finished, Angela and I were asked to leave the room while they voted. The two of us sat silently outside in the hallway, and I didn't want to move, as if any motion might affect the outcome.

I knew how pivotal this moment was and how, in just a few minutes, the course of my sons' future would be determined.

Finally I took a deep breath. "Do you think they liked it? They were so quiet."

Angela nodded, but I could tell she was as nervous as I was. Her son was nonverbal, as well, and struggled with extreme behaviors, just like Alie and Jamie. She needed this program as much as we did.

Then the door opened, and Angela and I walked back into the room and the Board Chair told us the vote for Genesis was unanimous. I wanted to hug each of those board members. For the first time in a long time, I felt my body relax.

As I was leaving that night, a parent member of the Board stopped me and reached for my hand. She cupped it in both of hers. "I was you years ago," she said. "My son, he's in his 20s now, and he's doing so well, but only because of Eden II." She told me how she and other families just like ours founded Eden II in 1976 with six children and one special education teacher. Since then, it had grown to serve over 300 children, adults, and their families each year.

In that moment, I knew we were part of something larger than ourselves, something that would not only make a difference in Alie and Jamie's lives, not only in Angela's, Ellen's, Sharon's, and Olga's children's lives, but in the lives of countless children with autism on Long Island for years to come.

"Thank you," I said, gratitude thick in my throat.

"No, thank *you*," she said, smiling. "Thank you for fighting for your sons. You're a special mom. They're lucky to have you."

I thought of the other moms fighting alongside me. I thought of my own mom, who had worked tirelessly for her students all those years and who would have done anything for my sister Edie and me. I nodded my thanks and hoped this school would be what would finally cure my sons—cure all of our children.

After the board meeting, everything moved quickly. Our "autism club" went into full gear. We searched for a school location and obtained donations of school supplies, furniture, and educational toys. Genesis, because it was providing special education at a level that mainstream schools could not provide, would also receive funding from each school district from which the students came. So Joanne worked on identifying other potential students to make the school financially sustainable for the first year.

Staff from all of our home programs were interested in working at the school, which was ideal because it would make the transition easier for everyone. Then Joanne called to tell me about Mary McDonald, who had been working as the Director of ABA services for QSAC (Quality Services for the Autism Community) in Queens. Joanne had met Mary at a few conferences and knew she was interested in someday being the director of a school for children with autism, so she had convinced Mary to apply to be the director of Genesis. Mary was hesitant because she had recently started a doctoral program in learning processes and she didn't feel ready to take the leap into running a school. But Joanne convinced her to at least meet some of the families.

I'll never forget the day I met Mary. She and Joanne came to my house, and we sat in the living room, in the same spot Joanne had trained our home staff the year before. Light poured in the back windows, and I could feel the hopeful energy in the room. I knew that if Joanne was recruiting Mary, she had to be good. And as Joanne rattled off Mary's experience and qualifications, I could tell how much she respected her.

Mary seemed serene as she sat there, and I wondered briefly if she had the drive to run a school like Genesis. But as she listened to me talk about Jamie and Alie and our home program, the progress they were making, and our plans for Genesis, her face transformed.

She tucked her long auburn hair behind her ear and leaned forward. Then she began talking about her work with children and families at QSAC and how exciting it was to be a part of that kind of learning.

"I have high hopes and expectations for all kids," she said, smiling. "That includes kids with autism. A school like Genesis can make a huge difference. There's so much we can do."

And I knew she was the one.

When Joanne called Mary the following week to see if she would accept the position, she said, her voice full of excitement, "Yes! I can't possibly turn this down."

––––

In September of 1995, when Alie and Jamie were five years old, Genesis opened as a two-room school in Plainview, Long Island. It was bare bones in those early days: six children, one teacher, and three assistants in each of two classrooms. And Mary. That was it. There was no secretary, no office staff, nothing. They had to hire a speech therapist hourly. But we had done it; we'd opened a school exclusively for children with autism on Long Island.

Shortly thereafter, Mary sent me a framed photograph of a rocket soaring over the moon into outer space. Under the photograph were the words "VISION" and the Carl Sandburg quote, "Nothing happens unless first a dream." But I understood that Genesis was not only my vision and not only the vision of the other parents who had worked so hard to make it happen. It was Joanne's vision and it was Mary's vision, as well. They wanted it just as much as I did. We were in it together, and I was so grateful.

––––

Having the boys in school all day created some breathing room in our lives. We still did intensive home therapy in the afternoons and on the weekends, but I had fewer discrete trial programs to transfer each night. Ruth and Randy were still working in the program, and

I relied on them more and more. At this point Ruth was overseeing the program, and I don't know what I would have done without her. She helped train new staff, and if I had a problem with a staff person, if I didn't feel they were responding correctly to the boys, Ruth would intervene. She was more diplomatic than I was, and she also had a calming effect on me. Somehow she could get me to slow down, at least for a moment, and breathe.

Because of their intense ABA therapy, the boys were now very responsive to direction, and their understanding of functional directions made a huge difference in our daily lives. We could tell Jamie to go get his sneakers, and he'd understand us and do it. Or we could tell Alie to turn off the light, and he would reach over and switch it off.

But we still worried about their safety. One of the scariest things for any parent, but especially for parents whose children have autism, is when their children wander off. Children with autism are four times more likely to wander off than their typical peers. This elopement accounts, in part, for the high rates of death for children with autism, rates that are almost double what they are for the general population. Both of the boys were prone to wandering off, but especially Jamie. We spent hours and hours teaching them to come when we called their names. And we hid Jamie all over the house and then called "Jamie, come here! Jamie, come here!" We practiced for months, and he finally learned to come to us when we called, no matter where he was.

———

We were making progress, but managing them was still a two-person, 24-hour-a-day job. They still got into everything, and they had no fear. If I left them alone in the kitchen, they would be up on the counters or table. They didn't understand to sit on a chair rather than stand on it. And even though they were five years old, they still had many toileting accidents. Their stereotypy was also still difficult to manage. Jamie still jumped, jumped, jumped. He did it happily, windmilling his arms, but still, it was disruptive. At least now when we told him to stop, he understood and would stop, but he'd start up again after a minute or two, so he still needed to be constantly monitored. Alie didn't respond as well when we asked him to stop tapping or flapping his arms. It was as if we couldn't break through the sensory field that surrounded him when he was absorbed in that kind of stimulatory movement. Sometimes one behavior would stop, but another one would pop up. It was like trying to control a forest fire. As soon as flames died down in one area, they would ignite somewhere else.

In the mornings, Allan and I would tag-team. Allan got breakfast ready as I got Jamie and Alie up and to the bathroom and dressed. He fed them while I got ready for work, and then he got ready for work as I cleaned them up and got them ready for school. As soon as the boys were on the bus, we'd both head out the door to work.

Work was stressful for me—I wished I could be home when the boys got home from school—and I no longer had the drive to move up the corporate ladder. But even with the assistance from the state, which paid for the home program and for home care assistance, we needed my income. This was especially true because Allan had decided to leave the real estate business. It had become unmanageable in the face of his MS attacks, which had begun to recur every few months and lasted for weeks. He was plagued by severe headaches, slurred speech, and leg cramps. And his debilitating fatigue still struck him every afternoon. His still owned the used car and repair business, so he decided to focus solely on that, which allowed him the flexibility to be home when the boys got home from school and to rest every afternoon.

Barbara, our nanny, had gone back to school to complete her degree in nursing, but we still needed the extra help, so we hired Marjorie, who was a godsend. She helped care for the boys in the afternoons until their therapists arrived, and she also helped with cooking and cleaning and other household tasks that I didn't have time to complete after the boys were asleep and after I had readied everything for the following day. Marjorie was a wonderful cook who had learned to prepare French food from her Haitian mother and grandmother, so we ate well during the years she was with us. Even the boys loved her cooking. She always had a huge, dimpled smile for me when I came in the door, and she loved the boys, never seeming bothered by their behaviors.

———

That first year that the boys were at Genesis was filled with hope. I felt they were finally somewhere they could thrive and recover. They had adapted to the new routine and they were learning. And at school they now had gym class, which they loved because they got to burn some of their frenetic energy.

Jamie, especially, seemed to be flourishing. We taught him the words to his favorite songs: the ABC Song, "Happy Birthday," "Bingo," "Old MacDonald Had a Farm," and Barney's "I Love You." He loved to sit on my lap facing me and sing and sing. His favorite was "Old MacDonald." I taught him to start with the cow, then the duck, then the dog, then the cat, and then the cow again. He would sing on and on, one animal after another, and I think he was very proud of himself, remembering the order of the animals so well. When he finished, I'd go crazy with reinforcement, holding him in the air and tickling him until he was belly laughing.

It was also a time of hope for Allan and me. Despite his recurring MS symptoms, we spent more time together, had nightly "debriefings" in which I'd fill him in on what was happening with the boys at school, and he would fill me in on what was happening in the world. Sometimes we'd cuddle and watch a movie. Occasionally, we'd have my mom and dad come over and we'd go out for dinner. It was a year of possibility, a year in which our hard work seemed to be paying off.

7

It's not uncommon for children with autism to rapidly acquire skills in the first months and years of intensive ABA work. But after that initial burst of skill acquisition, learning sometimes slows down or plateaus. I didn't know this when the boys were young. They had been learning so quickly, and now they had intensive ABA at school and at home. I expected them to keep making fast progress, advancing toward recovery.

I hadn't let go of the dream that Catherine Maurice planted in my mind when I read *Let Me Hear Your Voice*. Maurice's daughter, Anne-Marie, basically lost her diagnosis of autism within eight months of beginning intensive ABA. By two and a half, she had "moved into the clearly normal range of adaptive skills." She had started ABA earlier than Alie and Jamie, of course, but I had hoped that at five years old and with over a year and a half of ABA, they would be further along on the path to recovery. There wouldn't be as much stereotypy, not as many tantrums. I knew that every child with autism was different, and I tried to remind myself of that, tried to maintain hope. But I could feel it faltering.

———

When the boys were five-and-a-half years old, we took them down to Florida so we could spend a week with my parents in Boynton Beach, where they had settled in as "snow birds." When the boys were three, before we started our home program, I never would have dreamed of taking them on an airplane—of expecting them to transition from home to cab to airport to plane without an epic meltdown (or 10). And the thought of a plane full of strangers witnessing that kind of thing with horrified looks on their faces—well, it was too much to even contemplate.

But now they knew how to follow directions and they understood what was expected of them. In preparation for our trip I had, of course, spent hours on the phone with Delta, arranging early boarding and seats near the front of the plane in case we needed to exit quickly upon landing. And I packed a bag full of reinforcers and things to placate them: their CD players and favorite music, books, extra batteries, and headphones. And apples. Apples at this point worked magic. Whenever we needed to transition the boys from one place to the other, we handed them apples, and the taste, the tartness—who knew exactly what it was—somehow undercut the anxiety that transitions incited in them.

On Dr. Bergtraum's suggestion, we also gave each of the boys a dose of Benadryl before boarding the plane, which made them sleepy and compliant. Aside from Jamie leaping across the aisle into the lap of a woman in the window seat on the right side of the plane just before takeoff, we made it to Florida without incident. (We had been correct in thinking that Jamie would want the window seat so he could watch the landscape slip by below us, but we didn't realize he wanted the window on the *right* side of the plane rather than the left. Luckily the woman was very gracious, waved away our apologies, and switched seats with us.)

Allan and I both took deep, grateful breaths as we touched down at the Palm Beach airport, and we relaxed into days spent with my parents, who were thriving in their new community. They had been hesitant to make the move—to spend those winter months so far away from us each year, knowing they wouldn't be able to pop over and help with the boys each week or drive down and see Edie and her family where they now lived in Pennsylvania. But I knew the winters in New York were beginning to wear on them, and after all their years of hard work—Dad as the northeastern regional head of the IRS and Mom as a special education teacher—they deserved a little sun and golf. It was immediately clear that they had settled in. Mom was full of talk of this friend or that dinner party. I loved to see them happy.

And it *was* wonderful to have the extra help with Alie and Jamie. We even went out to dinner a couple of times, something we rarely did with Alie and Jamie in Great Neck because it was too difficult for Allan and me to eat our own dinner *and* contain the boys. Not to mention that other diners often seemed disturbed by the boys' whining screeches and flapping arms. But my dad insisted: "We all have a right to eat out." Their behavior in public never discomfited him; he was never flustered or irritated with them. He just laughed his infectious laugh and seemed to defuse any discomfort that surrounded us.

We spent the warm, sunny days holding Alie's and Jamie's hands as they dashed into the shallow waves. One day Mom and I sat on lounge chairs and watched as Allan raced up and down the beach with them. They squealed in delight, their laughter riding on the salty air. I shielded my eyes with my hand to see them more closely, and I thought, *They look like normal five-year-olds playing with their dad. But would they ever be "normal"? Would they ever recover fully from autism?* I gave myself a mental shake. *Don't think about that. They're doing well. They're happy.*

As if my mom could hear my thoughts, she said, "Look how happy they are! They love to run!"

I nodded, smiling. "They do." But I couldn't shake the sadness that had settled over me.

One morning, Dad and I took the boys to a playground. They were zooming through tunnels and flying down slides. They dove into the white sand and were up again, running, running, running. My dad and I sat on a bench, smiling as we watched them go.

I loved to just sit there next to Dad, watching Alie and Jamie. It reminded me of other times through the years that we sat next to each other, sharing an experience, not needing to talk. Once when I was about eight, Dad asked if I wanted to go to synagogue with him for Rosh Hashanah. Dad had been raised Orthodox and went to a more conservative synagogue than Mom and Edie and me. That day I remember feeling so proud as I sat next to him on the bench, even though I didn't understand any of the service because it was completely in Hebrew. I just sat there next to Dad, watching him, standing when he stood, sitting when he sat. Even as a child I understood he was offering me a gift, a way for us to be even more connected. So I sat as still as possible, letting the melodic intonations of Hebrew roll through me, letting the haunting sound of the shofar fill my chest.

At the park in Florida, I couldn't be that still. I was up and down, redirecting Alie and Jamie when they got stuck, Alie tapping his hand on the edge of the slide, Jamie jumping and jumping. When I settled myself back on the bench next to Dad after one such incident, he put his arm around me. I let myself relax into him, as I always did.

After a moment he said, quietly, "Robyn, at some point you're going to have to think about where the boys are going to end up, who will take care of them."

I didn't say anything in response. I watched the boys laughing as they flew down the slide and ran up the steps. Down the slide and up the steps. They were happy. They were just little kids. I wasn't ready to go there.

"Have you thought about it?" he prodded.

I hadn't, not really, but in that moment I finally understood that I would *need* to think about it. "I know," I said quietly, my eyes filling with tears.

Dad took my hand in his and he didn't say anything else. That's how he was—he didn't need to say much; he just planted a seed. I knew how much he loved me, knew how much he loved the boys, and I knew it broke his heart that they had autism. But he was also a realist, and he'd say what needed to be said: that Alie and Jamie most likely wouldn't be cured of autism, that they would probably always need help. This was long-term. This was our life.

———

Around the same time that I was beginning to acknowledge that the boys would probably never be cured of autism, Joanne was coming to a similar conclusion. She had worked with them closely for months and months, had watched them make quick progress in the beginning and then slow down. I didn't realize it then, but by the time they were five and a half years old, she knew the boys wouldn't recover from autism. Our team meetings at this point were suddenly no longer just about teaching strategies and new skill acquisition; we had to spend more and more time focused on emerging behaviors that were interfering with their learning.

Both boys had started to show signs of increased anxiety and obsessive-compulsive disorder (OCD). OCD is characterized by intrusive thoughts that cause distress and repeated behaviors that someone suffering from OCD performs again and again and again to try to assuage the anxiety caused by the obsessions. Alie couldn't tolerate any changes in his schedule. If the day didn't unfold exactly how he expected it would (and how it had the day before), his agitation would lead to grabbing or biting. And though Alie couldn't tell time, he had an inner clock and knew exactly when therapy sessions were supposed to be over or when it was time for lunch or a shower or bed. When things didn't happen exactly when his clock dictated, he'd become distraught and begin stomping his feet on the hardwood floor. Jamie's compulsions were more subtle; he would tap a certain spot on the front stoop every day, and shut any open door, spellbound by the movement of its closing. If we interrupted him as he tapped or shut doors, he would spin out into a tantrum.

Years later Joanne would explain to me that the children who recover from autism are the ones who don't have comorbid neurological disorders. Jamie and Alie, it was becoming clear, *did* have comorbid neurological disorders: they were obsessive-compulsive, had high levels of anxiety, and they were, to some degree, intellectually disabled. Those issues can't be fixed with ABA. All you can do is work around them, to focus on improving the symptoms of autism *despite* the coexisting neurological limitations.

At that point I didn't understand that their underlying neurological issues were a roadblock to recovery. And I guess it wouldn't have mattered anyway. That realization wouldn't have stopped me from doing everything I could for them. There had already occurred in me a subtle shift, a slight turning away from focusing on their cure and recovery to focusing on their happiness. How, if they would never recover from autism, could I ensure that their lives would be full of joy?

In the years after that trip to Florida, I kept pushing forward, trying to make sure Alie and Jamie were learning as much as they could. We continued to juggle school and the home program. But in an effort to find the things that made the boys happy, Allan and I also enrolled them in as many activities as possible, chasing after the things that we could see they enjoyed.

We signed them up for horseback riding, soccer, karate, and swimming—anything that would allow them to participate in activities that typical kids their age enjoyed. Some of these activities were more successful than others. They loved swimming lessons at our local Jewish community center. When we told Jamie that we were going to go swimming, he'd begin to vocalize happily and jump, his arms spinning through the air. The boys had one-to-one swimming instruction with a gentle teacher, who, though he knew nothing about autism, seemed to "get" the boys. Jamie, especially, was enthralled with the teacher's hair, which swayed back and forth in a long dark ponytail. I was afraid they'd end up at the bottom of the pool, but instead they paddled around with their floaty armbands, slapping the water and giggling. Swimming became a powerful reinforcer over the years.

They also loved horseback riding and were calmed by those large, gentle creatures. I had loved riding when I was growing up as well, and I had spent hours every week brushing the horses at the stable where I took lessons. I understood the horses' calming effect, and I loved to watch Alie and Jamie smiling as they were trotted around the large corral on a long lead.

Soccer and karate were less successful. In karate class, they had to sit for long periods of time, which was never easy for either of them. And soccer was a disaster. Even though it was a program specifically for children with special needs, neither Alie nor Jamie understood what was expected of them. There were too many rules, too much foot coordination. And at that point, they weren't fast enough to steal the ball from their opponents.

One of our home therapists, Janine, owned a gymnastics center with her husband, and she suggested we bring the boys in to see if they might like it. Alie and Jamie's eyes lit up at all the climbing equipment, so Janine began giving them one-to-one lessons. They learned the balance beam, the high bar, the ropes, the horse, and the trampoline—everything that typical kids learn in gymnastics. For years we went every Sunday morning for an hour-long lesson, and the boys loved it. Janine was bubbly and positive, always convinced that the boys could master the activity at hand. They seemed to understand when they had executed one of the exercises correctly, because they would beam. They even waited patiently for their turn.

At the end of that first year, Janine insisted that the boys compete in the annual show, even though it was for neurotypical gymnasts. I'll never forget that day. We sat on folding chairs with other parents. There were competitions going on throughout the gymnasium, and when one of the other gymnasts executed a perfect dismount or made their bodies weightless, flipping through the air, loud cheers erupted around us. Allan and I cheered loudly for the boys when they performed, even though their routines were elementary. The parents surrounding us must have realized that the boys had special needs because they, too, were soon cheering loudly, screaming their encouragement, for which I was grateful. At the end of the competition, Janine held the boys' hands, and she triumphantly raised their arms in the air with hers. Alie and Jamie were glowing, and Allan and I were both in tears.

8

WHAT WE LEARNED IN THE following years is that every day with twins who have severe autism is different—behaviors that are problematic one day are sometimes gone the next day, only to be replaced with new problematic behavior the following day. It was exhausting, trying to stay a step ahead of that constant changing. But how can you stay a step ahead of it if you don't even know what "it" will look like?

During those first years at Genesis, Jamie was still calmer than Alie, but he was erupting more frequently with noncontextual vocalizations, humming, and garbled singing, and he continued to bend his fingers backward against desks and tables so hard that we were afraid he'd break or dislocate them. Pain didn't register.

Pica was still a huge problem for Alie—I would often catch him with thread or paper in his mouth—and, like Jamie, he still engaged in lots of stereotypy: flapping his hands and snapping his wrists. We worried that Alie, too, might break a bone because he would snap his wrists so forcefully and frequently. Alie was also developing more aggressive behaviors: when he was upset, he'd kick, grab, bite, and hit—both himself and others.

These increasing behavioral problems seemed to stem, at least in part, from the fact that the boys still hadn't developed enough functional expressive language to really communicate with others. Jamie had more intelligible verbal language than Alie; he could say approximately 100 words. But he didn't use these words spontaneously. He had echolalia, so he would imitate words or, when prompted, read them from index cards. Both boys could read simple words, so we taped index cards all over the house labeling everything—door, light, chair, TV, table, bed—to try to get them to use the words they knew, but they never did unless prompted. Jamie was able to respond to a yes or no question, or if we asked "What do you want?" and he knew the word for what he wanted, he would reply with it. He was also able to say, "tickle me," which was one of his big reinforcers. He would laugh so hard and seem so happy that it was hard to stop tickling him.

Alie hadn't developed much verbal expressive language at all, so with him we began using a Picture Exchange Communication System (PECS), a Velcro board with pictures on it meant to promote communication. We taught Alie that if he wanted a slice of apple, he had to hand us the picture with the apple on it. After he mastered exchanging a picture for an object he wanted, we added the words "I want" to a square and taught him how to put the picture of whatever he wanted next to "I want" to create a sentence. Alie picked it up quickly, so after a few months he advanced to using an augmentative and alternative communication (AAC) device, which had a touch screen with pictures. When Alie pressed the picture of an apple on his screen, a programmed voice would say "apple." We would wait until Alie repeated the word before his request would be granted, which forced him to verbalize. Having that ability to ask for what he wanted alleviated some of Alie's distress, but he still couldn't tell us how he was feeling. Neither of the boys could tell us if they were upset or angry or hurt. They couldn't articulate emotion. And that inability to communicate how they were feeling or what was upsetting them led to more severe behaviors.

———

In January 1998, when the boys were seven years old, my dad was celebrating his 80th birthday, and he and my mom had hoped that we would be able to bring the boys down for the party. (It was technically a surprise party, but Dad knew all about it, and he couldn't contain his glee at the prospect of having his closest friends gathered together to celebrate his special day. He gloated for months about joining the ranks of octogenarians.) But there was no way we could take the boys down to Florida at this point; their problem behaviors had become too unpredictable. There was also no way we could go without them. We could have lined up therapists to take care of them around the clock, but neither Allan nor I felt comfortable leaving them at home while we jetted off to Florida for a party. So we decided not to go.

But one morning before work, Allan sat me down at the kitchen table. "Robyn, you have to go to your dad's party." His voice was stern, his hands splayed in the air. "I'll stay here with the boys. I'll have plenty of help."

My first reaction was, *No way. There is no way I'm leaving the boys.* The only time I'd been away from them for a night was when they were infants. My parents stayed with them while Allan and I spent a night at a hotel to celebrate our anniversary. But that was before their diagnosis, before autism. Now I couldn't imagine leaving Allan to deal with them on his own, especially with their escalating behaviors. They were at least a two-person job.

But Allan kept pressing me. "Rob, we'll be fine. You have to go. You know how much it will mean to your parents. Besides, Ruth will be on call." Allan had made up his mind, and I could tell he wasn't going to back down.

I'm surprised that with everything that was going on with the boys, I listened to Allan. But I'm so grateful I did. My parents were radiant that weekend, surrounded by so many of their friends. Part of me felt guilty, of course, and I called home to check on the boys several times a day. But part of me felt so free being there on my own.

I didn't have to constantly monitor the boys. I didn't have to watch for signs of burgeoning distress. I didn't have to redirect anyone or put out any fires. And each time I got a good report from Allan, I relaxed a little more, allowing Dad's joy to rub off on me. The day of the party, every time the phone rang, Dad would rush to pick it up. "Hello hello hello!" he'd exclaim in his singsong voice. "Happy Surprise Birthday to me!"

Mom and I just laughed and shook our heads.

That night, Dad stood at the door, welcoming his friends with hugs and thanking them for coming to his surprise party.

———

It was the last time I saw him. On April 3 Mom left a message on our home answering machine: "Allan, it's Mom. Please call me when you get this message." It was early afternoon, so Allan should have heard the message first, but that day Jamie wasn't feeling well, so I had to leave work and pick him up at school. When I returned home and listened to the message, I knew something was wrong. Mom sounded composed but off. I settled Jamie in the den to watch *Sesame Street* and then picked up the phone to call Mom. My hands were shaking as I dialed her number. No answer. So I dialed her friend Bea's number. Again no answer.

I somehow knew that something was terribly wrong. Something had happened to Dad. I called information and got the numbers for JFK and Bethesda Hospitals, two hospitals in Boynton Beach. I called JFK and asked if Dad had been brought in. No. Momentary relief. Then I called Bethesda, and they said yes. I asked for more information and was put on hold. My whole body was trembling. *He's going to be fine. He's going to be fine.* From the other room I could hear the high-pitched voices of Ernie and Bert.

Finally a doctor came on the line and I explained who I was. "What happened? How is my dad?"

"I'm so sorry to have to tell you this," the doctor said slowly. "But your father has passed away." I couldn't breathe. *He couldn't have died. I just saw him. He was so happy. He can't be gone.* I don't remember what I said to the doctor, if anything. My skin had turned to ice. Later I learned that he had a heart attack while he was playing chess with a friend at the clubhouse. By the time the ambulance arrived at the hospital, he was gone.

———

It was only after Dad died that I understood the extent to which he had been advocating on Alie and Jamie's behalf. That summer, as I was helping Mom go through his study in their house in East Meadow, I found files and files of articles about autism, pages filled with notes he had taken while talking to experts around the country. As I stood there in my parents' house, surrounded by all those papers, the evidence of his love for my family and me, I was overcome with grief. What would I do without him?

I was also frightened that my mother would die, if not from grief—my parents had been married 56 years—then from something else. I worried about her constantly, but tried to put on a happy face for her because I knew she was devastated. But I also couldn't shake my own grief. Dad's death left a huge void in our lives. Everything seemed more arduous without his infectious laughter and unyielding support.

All of this made Alie's blossoming aggression even more difficult to bear. I was often called into meetings at Genesis with Mary, his teachers, and the rest of the team. They would conduct a functional assessment to determine what was causing his aggression and self-injurious behavior.

"Alie is focused and persistent," Mary said. "His behavior is goal-oriented, even though it may not seem functional to everyone else." It was investigative work to try to get to the root of why certain behaviors were happening, to understand Alie's goal. But very often, the reasons weren't clear. Was he seeking attention? Or was there something physical going on? Or worse, neurological? Why was he so upset so often?

After reviewing all the data that was collected by school and home staff, Mary would develop a plan to address the behaviors and start applying interventions. The philosophy at Genesis had always been to develop and implement behavior plans that proactively addressed problem behavior without physical intervention. But in order to keep Alie from hurting himself or someone else, they had to include in his plan an option for physical restraint. It made me sick to think of him having to be restrained. But I also knew that this would only occur if all else failed.

Allan and I needed to learn how to restrain him when he was out of control at home, as well. Mary and Randy, who by then had been promoted to the Director of Educational Services for Eden II and Genesis, urged us to attend a special parent training at the school on Strategies for Crisis Intervention and Prevention (SCIP).

I never imagined that the boys' autism would get that bad. I never imagined that one day Allan and I would be sitting in a room full of other heartbroken parents, all of us learning blocking and holding techniques to use on our own children. The devastation of the boys' diagnosis paled in comparison with the knowledge that someday I might need to restrain Alie with my own hands, hands that had fed him and Jamie, hands that rocked them, hands that held them to my chest. How could I do that with my own body, a body that had grown and nurtured my sons?

Allan and I both felt better attending the training, though, knowing that we'd be prepared if we needed to restrain Alie at home. But even as we sat there, watching and practicing technique after technique, I refused to let myself believe we'd ever need to do it. Somehow

Alie would snap out of his new aggressive patterns. Somehow he would turn a corner.

This was, perhaps, one of the most agonizing aspects of the boys' autism for me, the way we couldn't count on anything to stay the same. We couldn't count on the boys sustaining the progress that they'd made. We couldn't count on things not suddenly getting worse. We could never be complacent.

———

Around this time, when the boys were almost 10, Ruth and I had taken Alie to Dr. Bergtraum to talk about his increased aggression. Dr. Bergtraum suggested a mood stabilizer. Allan and I were both resistant to medication because of the side effects. A couple of months earlier, on the recommendation of a psychiatrist, we had tried Alie on Risperdal, an antipsychotic. Allan and I were stunned by the recommendation—an antipsychotic?—but because his aggression was so problematic, we tried it. Alie was up all night, every night. None of us slept for a week, so we took him off it. The last thing we needed was another week without sleep, or something worse. Allan, in particular, was adamantly opposed to medicating the boys. The side effects— extreme headaches and fatigue—of the medication that he had been prescribed after his diagnosis with MS were more debilitating than the symptoms of the disease. What if this was the case with Alie? He wouldn't even be able to tell us how he felt.

Like Randy and Mary and Joanne, Ruth was a rock for me. They were all experts at what they did, but more importantly, they had all grown into friends, friends who loved Alie and Jamie. I knew they always had the boys' best interests at heart. Ruth, especially, had a way of grounding me. I was grateful that she had accompanied me to the appointment. On the drive home, we talked about Dr. Bergtraum's recommendations.

"I don't know," I said. "I know Allan is going to say that we're just doping him up, but this isn't Risperdal, and we have to do something."

Ruth was quiet for a moment, and I knew she was thinking how best to phrase her next statement. That's how she was, always thoughtful. She also knew me well enough to know how to present information so that I could really "hear" it. Finally she said, "I know you and Allan are worried about the side effects of medicating Alie. I really understand that. But Alie's whole life is becoming a side effect. Robyn, he's suffering."

I just nodded, letting her words sink in.

We arrived home in the early afternoon, and it didn't even occur to me that this might be a problem for Alie. I should have known. Alie was extremely dependent on routines. His internal clock had become ultraprecise. He knew exactly when it was time to wake up and leave for school. He knew what time the home therapists would arrive and exactly when they should leave. (He would gather their bags or keys the minute the session was scheduled to end.) If dinner was even five minutes late, the dam would break and his anxiety would spill out.

That day it was a school day, but he wasn't in school. He was home "too early," but Jamie wasn't there with him. We thought it would be okay, though. Ruth set him up in the den with his activity schedule. It was hard for Alie to sit still and focus. He wanted to move all the time. But he liked starting a task and ending a task, so we developed activity schedules for him that consisted of pictures of games, books, and puzzles on Velcro boards. He would point to the picture at the top of the schedule, then go get the actual activity or game and play it. Once he was done with that activity, he took the corresponding picture off and moved on to the next picture. This would sometimes keep him busy for an hour.

Ruth and I started moving into the living room to continue talking about Alie's appointment. But suddenly, Alie was no longer on the floor playing. He was coming toward me, his arms out. He was vocalizing loudly, unintelligibly, his face contorted in distress. It looked like he was going to attack me, but I was more shocked than scared. He'd never done anything like that before.

"Alie, Alie," said Ruth. "Alie, time to go back to your schedule." She tried to redirect him.

But it was as if he couldn't hear her. He spun around and made a beeline for Ruth, his hands curled in the air as if he was going to scratch her face or eyes. He was just a kid, but he was strong. He kept reaching toward Ruth.

"Hands down, Alie. Hands down." She moved his hands to his sides. "Alie, look at this." She held up the CD player, the reinforcer he was to get after he finished his activities. "Alie, do you want to listen to music?" But nothing worked—he was suddenly in a frenzy, trying to scratch Ruth's arms, her face. Everything blurred in front of me. Alie twirling. Ruth reaching for him. Turn, twist. Alie in SCIP. Ruth's arms wrapped over Alie's, crisscross over his chest. Alie thrashing, trying to bite her.

It all happened so fast, but it was as if I was watching the whole thing unfold in slow motion. Then Alie dropped to the floor, and Ruth went down with him. He was flailing around on the floor and Ruth was holding on tight.

I glanced down at my hands, which were shaking. Tears streamed down my face. *How could this be my son? What is happening to him? Why? How can we stop him?*

But Alie was unstoppable. He was screeching, throwing back his head, trying to head-butt Ruth, trying to wiggle from her grasp. How long did it go on? I don't know. It was as if we were suspended in time, cemented in one horrible moment, unable to break free.

Alie finally stopped thrashing, his body releasing some of the intense rigidity, and Ruth was able to let him go. He was sweating and pale. I wiped away my tears with the back of my hand and got up to get him a cup of water.

We finally got him settled in front of the TV and turned on *Barney*, which he still loved, and Ruth and I sat down at the kitchen table. We were both pale. All of Ruth's usual vivaciousness was gone. I was so relieved that Marjorie wasn't working that day and hadn't had to witness Alie like that. It would have broken her heart.

She reached for my hand. "Robyn, he's okay. He's safe."

I nodded. He was safe now, thanks to her. I hoped Ruth understood how grateful I was that she had been there, that she was there now. But why had it happened? What had flipped that switch in him? We tried to piece together what had triggered Alie, but all we could come up with was the change in his routine.

Ruth would later tell me that that day was the beginning of a critical understanding for her as a teacher and therapist working with kids with severe autism. "So many of 'our kids' can be a certain and predictable way," she'd tell me. "But there are factors, both environmental and medical, that can grossly alter what we think we know or what we once knew about them."

I don't know if I consciously tried to erase that day from memory or if it was automatic self-preservation that buried it deep in my mind. I just couldn't permit that kind of suffering to take hold of me. I didn't want to remember Alie like that, flying at us with his hands raised, even if that was our reality. It was only years later, when Ruth and I were talking about that day, that the details came flooding back.

It's not surprising that studies have shown that mothers of children and adolescents with autism have stress levels similar to combat soldiers. Like soldiers, autism moms have low levels of cortisol, which is an indicator of chronic stress. Other studies have pointed to the high rate of post-traumatic stress disorder (PTSD) in autism moms. I understand that. I remember the stress of every single day not knowing how the day would unravel, if Alie would hurt himself, if Jamie would see and hear Alie melting down and become scared and agitated himself. Some days it felt as though we lived on a battlefield. It was hard enough having two sons with autism, but the intensity and danger of these new behaviors—sometimes it felt like too much to bear.

———

If Alie was going through a crisis period, which was happening more and more, Ruth would spend extra time with us at home to help Allan and me manage his behaviors, but she couldn't be there all the time. When Allan or I had to do a SCIP hold on Alie, we'd get him to the floor with one of us sitting behind him and wrap Alie's arms across his chest with our arms over his, as Ruth had done. The few times I had to do this at home, I sat there holding him, dodging his bites, crying. We were trying to do everything right, carefully following all his behavior plans, and still, we would end up on the floor with him, our arms wrapped tightly around him, trying to keep him and ourselves safe.

Because Alie's tantrums set off Jamie, Allan and I both tried to spend time separately with Jamie away from home. Jamie loved to be out and about. Sometimes we'd go out for ice cream, other times to the park or the bookstore. One day when I took him to the bookstore, there was a little girl with a blond ponytail in the next aisle. Jamie was captivated. Was it her swaying ponytail? Her smile? Or just the fact that she was another kid looking at books with her mother? I don't know, but when I glanced at the shelf to return the book I was holding, Jamie walked over to her and held out his hand to shake hers. Her mom tilted her head, puzzled. It certainly wasn't the behavior of a typical 10-year-old boy.

When I explained that Jamie had autism and that he just wanted to shake her daughter's hand, the mom smiled and so did the little girl, holding her hand out for Jamie to grasp. I smiled, too, grateful to both of them. That's how Jamie was, just wanting to connect with people. But then we would return home, and if Alie was upset, Jamie would instantly pick up on it and spiral out of control, as well.

There were months during these years when I felt like I was watching the clock all afternoon and evening, counting the hours, hoping it would be a day free of major incidents. Even as I sat at my desk at work, the boys were always on my mind. *Please let their day be going okay. Please no dangerous behaviors today.*

I know my dad wouldn't have been able to do anything to improve things for us, but he would have tried. And, maybe more importantly, he would have just been there, like a buoy, helping to keep me afloat.

———

Not long after our appointment with Dr. Bergtraum, I was in the kitchen putting dishes away while Allan was with the boys in the den. Then Alie ran into the kitchen and was clearly agitated, squeezing and scratching his hands, biting his arms. I handed him his AAC device and asked him what he wanted, but he swatted it away from me. He lurched around the kitchen and pulled on my arm, and I could see he was working himself up. I put down the plate I was holding. "Alie, Alie, look at me." His face contorted as he raked his nails down my arm.

I felt the sudden sting of pain. My stomach dropped. "Alie, it's okay." I tried to hand him his AAC device again, and he hit it away, sending it clattering across the floor.

"Alie. Alie."

But nothing worked. Then he was suddenly a twirling mass of arms and legs.

I had done SCIP before and I knew I should be in a safe place, seated, before trying to restrain him, but I panicked. I bent down, grabbed his arms, and tried to wrap them across his chest. But Alie was like a trapped animal. He whipped his head back hard, and because I was leaning over him, his skull smashed into my mouth. Pain ricocheted across my face, radiating through my jaw. I must have screamed because Allan was suddenly there, yelling, "What happened? Oh my God, what happened?"

I had somehow slid to the kitchen floor without losing my hold on Alie, who was still thrashing, craning to try to bite me. I couldn't let Allan take over; that would just get Alie even more riled up, so I just held him tightly, crying into his hair, my mouth throbbing in pain.

When Alie finally went limp in my arms and I transferred him to Allan, I went into the bathroom, splashed water on my face, and stared at myself in the mirror. My lip was split, blood trickling down my chin. *How could this be our life? How did we get to this place? How will we find our way out of here?*

Rage and grief and heartbreak swirled through me, filling me up. I felt like throwing the mirror to the floor. *It's not fair!* I wanted to scream. But just as quickly, all that emotion drained away. This wasn't Alie's fault. This was intense and debilitating anxiety. This was autism.

Later that night, when Allan and I were lying in bed, I'm sure both of us looked shell-shocked. For a long time we just lay there, staring straight ahead, me with an ice pack pressed to my mouth.

"It's one thing after another," Allan finally said. "Rob, it's just too much for us to handle. And Alie's behavior is affecting Jamie."

"I know," I said. We'd never had to restrain Jamie, but what if that was next? Suddenly the tears came again, sadness spreading through my body.

Whenever I felt defeated about the boys, about what they (and we) were going through, I'd turn to Ruth or Randy or Mary or Joanne. They had seen so many other families battling autism, and I knew they could offer support, give me strength to keep fighting. Or I'd think of my parents, knowing that they would never give up. I had to stay strong, to keep going. But although Allan was involved in some of these conversations and meetings about the boys, he was largely processing the hard stuff on his own. His mother and siblings lived in Minnesota. He'd talk to them about it and occasionally to friends, but none of them really understood autism. They didn't understand what we were up against on a day-to-day basis. That isolation was wearing him down.

But that night, we were both utterly worn down. It was clear that we needed to do something different with Alie. Anxiety had taken hold and it was devouring him. Dr. Bergtraum had suggested medication might help, and that night, as Allan and I lay side by side, broken and exhausted, we realized it was time. Maybe it was past time.

9

EVEN THOUGH OUR LIVES WERE often characterized by chaos, and we had to put our heads down and just do what needed to be done to get through each day and each new crisis, we also experienced short periods of calm. During those moments, Allan and I slowed down a little and cautiously let joy seep into our lives. In the months after Alie went on medication, we experienced more of those moments than we had in a long time. Though Allan and I had been hesitant to medicate him, we knew we'd done the right thing when his extreme anxiety, and thus his self-injury and aggression, dissipated.

We still had to monitor both boys closely, making sure that we could nip new behaviors in the bud. But Alie was more relaxed, and as a result, so was Jamie. In the afternoon, Jamie loved to snuggle up to his favorite home therapists, and in the evenings, with Allan and me. After dinner, he would lie on the couch with his feet up on my lap, watching me with a smile on his face, waiting in anticipation for tickles.

Our evenings had moments of quiet. Marjorie had left to take a position working in a doctor's office closer to her home, and we were so sad to see her go. I knew we'd miss her amazing French cooking, but I'd also miss her dimpled smile. I knew, however, that we would always stay in touch with one another.

That winter we were able to take the boys to Disney World and visit my mom, who was still spending her winters in Florida. They loved the rides, loved the sensory explosion of barreling down the steep hills of the roller coaster or being pressed against the vinyl seats as they flew wildly through the air, strapped into swings that rose higher and higher into the blue sky. We had taken them to Disney World when they were younger, and it only took one visit for them to memorize where their favorite rides were, so this time, Allan and I were dragged from one side of the park to the other all day. But it was worth it to see their smiles.

Mom was still grieving for Dad, but like always, she tried to hide her pain from me. She had contemplated not returning to Florida, but Edie and I insisted, knowing that her community of friends in Boynton Beach would rally around her and make sure she got out of the house and enjoyed herself, which is exactly what they did.

And she was doing well, despite having to fight breast cancer just months after Dad died. Her cancer diagnosis had felt like a cruel joke. The thought that I might lose her after just losing Dad terrified me. How would I manage my life and the boys, without her strength too?

After her diagnosis, either Allan or I went to every doctor appointment with her, brought her meals, and called to check on her multiple times a day. Luckily, she didn't need chemotherapy, only radiation, but I cleared my schedule each week to make sure I could drive her to the radiology office and back and sit with her during each treatment. And Edie drove up from Pennsylvania each weekend to make sure Mom was never alone.

But though Mom's health was stable and she seemed happy surrounded by friends, both in Florida and when she was home in East Meadow, she was beginning to look more frail, and I worried about her more and more. Each morning on my way to work, I called just to hear her voice, just to make sure she was okay.

When Mom was in New York, Allan and I would often take her out for lunch, and I took her shopping each week. When she returned from Florida every spring, she loved to take drives to see the pink tulips and violet irises and yellow daffodils blooming in the expansive and elaborate gardens in nearby towns. And each fall, she'd exclaim over the delicious crisp air and the flaming oranges and deep reds of the changing leaves. I rarely noticed the colors around me. I never stopped to gaze up at the sky or marvel at the deepness of its blue. I never let myself get lost in the beauty of speckled sunlight through the maple trees that lined the road. I only had a couple of hours to run errands in the late afternoon while the boys were in home therapy, so I was always focused on the next thing on my list. But Mom's optimism and delight in what surrounded her was contagious. As she pointed out a bed of deep purple mums or an especially brilliant tree, I could feel myself being pulled from my protective shell. She could magically open the world for me to see.

On Father's Day, 2004, when my mom was 84 and the boys were 14 years old, I picked her up to take her to our house for a barbeque. As we drove down Shelter Rock Road toward my house, she gasped at the line of cherry trees, which were in full bloom. "Look how beautiful they are!" she exclaimed, and I smiled.

"They are, aren't they?" And it was as if I saw them for the first time, those snowy blossoms frothing into the early summer air.

At home, Allan and the boys were in the backyard. Alie and Jamie were jumping and running, jumping and running, while Allan put chicken on the grill. The boys were doing moderately well at school and at home. They were no longer taking gymnastics, but they still loved swimming and horseback riding lessons. Allan and I had also signed them up for the Police Academy League (PAL) basketball league for kids with special needs. The team was made up of adolescents with varied disabilities, and I always felt such pride as I watched their games—not just for Alie and Jamie, but for all the kids who were out there pushing themselves and having fun despite their limitations. Alie was really good at it, making nine out of ten baskets, and Jamie enjoyed the social aspect of being part of a team. He loved being patted on the back and getting high fives from his teammates. And both boys loved running back and forth on the court. We had come a long way from the days at the park when they were four and five years old. The other kids on the team weren't scared of my sons. The other parents didn't retreat from their differences. Here the boys—and Allan and I—were welcomed. And as I watched all the boys run up and down the court, I was reminded of how capable they were, how much they could accomplish despite the roadblocks in their way.

There were crises, of course, explosions of self-injurious behavior or new obsessions, but we were able to manage these with help from our teams at home and Genesis. Alie had stopped grabbing, scratching, and squeezing himself, but he started to bite his knuckles and nails. And he had begun to close his eyes while walking, which led to other accidents and injuries. Jamie still vocalized loudly and had begun to twist and rip his clothing. With his pinky finger he would rub at his jeans until he created a small tear that, throughout the day, would grow larger and larger. I patched some of his jeans, but often the holes were too big, and I just had to buy new ones. When he was agitated, he'd scratch or bite his hands, leaving red welts across his knuckles. They both remained on a structured 24/7 behavioral plan to keep things from escalating, and I still spent hours each night reviewing their data and writing detailed messages to their teachers and therapists about different approaches we might try. But for the most part, they—we—were doing okay.

On Father's Day, I was in and out of the house bringing things out to the patio for our lunch. Mom was sitting in the den reading the newspaper when I suggested she go outside, as well. Lunch was almost ready, and I wanted her to see the garden that Allan had just planted.

I held Mom's arm as we walked down the steps, but somehow she lost her balance, and we both went down, falling hard on the brick patio. I quickly jumped up, unhurt, but Mom just lay on the ground. "Mom!" I cried, and a chill shot through me, settling like ice in my veins.

Then everything was moving fast. Allan ran inside to call 911. I sat next to Mom on the ground, slipping a folded towel under her head.

"I'm okay. Don't worry." She smiled that same reassuring smile I'd seen a million times.

"Does anything hurt?" The sun suddenly was too bright, the air too humid. I could tell Mom was in pain, even though she was smiling.

"My leg hurts a little," she said, bringing a shaky hand to her forehead. "But I'm sure it will be okay."

The boys, still running and jumping, seemed oblivious to what had just happened. But then Jamie came over and reached out to touch Mom. I panicked, thinking he might try to pull her up and accidentally do more damage than the fall had already done. "No! No, Jamie!"

He flinched at the harshness in my voice, and immediately I felt horrible. He didn't understand why Grandma was on the ground. She wasn't supposed to be on the ground. He was just trying to help. I steadied my voice. "It's okay, Jamie. It's okay. Grandma just needs to stay where she is." Then I turned to Mom. "It's going to be okay, Mom. It's going to be okay." I didn't want to scare her or further scare Jamie.

As the paramedics lifted Mom on a stretcher into the ambulance, Allan squeezed my arm and gave me a quick hug. "Call me as soon as you know anything." He loved my parents as much as I did, and I knew he was worried. It was written all over his face.

I followed the ambulance in my car, wishing, willing the whole way: *she's going to be okay. Everything is going to be okay.*

At the hospital, X-rays confirmed a broken hip, which I'd feared. She had been in fairly good health, though, so I was hopeful that she'd recover quickly from any surgery she might need and be back home in a week or so. But once at the hospital, the doctors said she also needed heart bypass surgery. Suddenly her condition escalated, and after the bypass, one complication followed another and she ended up in intensive care. What we hoped would be a weeklong stay morphed into months.

For most of that time, I refused to believe anything except that she'd recover and be home soon: by the Fourth of July, by the beginning of August, by September, certainly by Halloween. After each setback she would rally, and the doctors would talk about rehab. I visited rehab facilities in the area, looking for the right place for her to do physical therapy and regain her strength before returning home. But she was 84, and her body just wasn't strong enough.

Those months were a complete blur. I was still up late every night trying to manage the boys' continually changing needs and address issues that arose at school and in the home program. I knew I couldn't manage home and the boys and be an advocate for Mom. My company was in the midst of restructuring, so it wasn't the best time for me to take time off, but Mom was my priority, so I decided to take FLMA leave so I could be with Mom at the hospital.

Thank God for Theresa, who had been working for us for a couple of years. Theresa was one of the kindest people I'd ever met. And nothing riled her. Over the years when Alie or Jamie had a tantrum or went through a period of especially intense OCD rituals, Theresa remained calm and avoided getting in the way. I knew she was there to support us any way she could, and I was grateful to have her calming presence at home while I was at the hospital with Mom.

I drove back and forth to the hospital three times a day to bring her things that might make her more comfortable: body lotion, magazines, newspapers, note cards and pens so she could write to her friends. I brought pictures of the boys and put them up on the walls. And I took over her bills and managing her house. Allan visited her every day, as well, and Edie and her husband Larry drove up from Pennsylvania every weekend, which was a relief because it was more difficult for me to spend long periods of time with her when the boys were at home. I could relax a little knowing that Edie and Larry and their sons Eric and Richard were there with her. But still I was feeling frazzled, and I could tell that juggling her hospitalization and the boys' behaviors was wearing on me. I snapped more often at Allan and was edgy and exasperated trying to stay ahead of the boys' behaviors.

Even with all the setbacks, Mom never complained. She remained positive until the last weeks when she became less and less aware of her surroundings and spent more and more time sleeping. I was with her, holding her hand, when she died on November 6, 2004. I thought I would be prepared—I knew it was only a matter of time at the end—but I wasn't at all. I felt shattered. I sat there next to her hospital bed, her hands in mine, my head on her bed, weeping. It didn't matter that I was a grown woman; I suddenly felt orphaned, abandoned. I lost my mom, and it was as if losing her made the grief over my dad grow stronger again. I was reeling for months.

———

After the funeral there were all of the details to deal with: the house, the condo, all their belongings, their finances. It was overwhelming. Perhaps it was a blessing that the restructuring at my job made it clear that I was no longer a fit for them, nor them for me. Between managing my parents' affairs and the boys, I didn't have time to work full time anyway. And it was never clearer that family was the priority— I wanted to spend as much time with Allan and the boys as possible. Even though I was by that point a vice president in the company, I resigned.

During these months of mourning, the boys kept me busy, as did the huge job of finalizing my parents' affairs. I was grateful that I didn't have to dash off every morning to a job that had lost its meaning for me. Thankfully, the money that Edie and I each inherited would make it possible for me to take time off from work and then find another job when things settled down.

Edie and I flew down to Florida to go through my parents' condo. Then both of us flew back to New York to begin the huge job of going through their home in East Meadow. The two of us hadn't spent much sustained time together since we were young. Edie was seven years older than I, so by the time I was 11, she was off to college, living her own life. Later, she and her family had moved several times for Larry's job, and because of the challanges traveling with the boys, we rarely visited them. But when I was young, I idolized her. I remember when she was 12 and I was five and she was leaving for sleep-away camp in Connecticut for the first time. She was going to be gone the whole summer, and I was devastated. I watched her pack her suitcase, wishing I could tuck myself in it, fold myself between the layers of her clothes. The day she left, my dad took a picture of us on the front steps. In the photo, her long blond hair is pulled into a sleek ponytail and she holds her valise in one hand and my hand in the other. She's smiling broadly into the camera. I have dark curly hair, Shirley Temple style, and I'm gazing up at her, a lump in my throat.

After Mom died, the only silver lining was that Edie and I were able to spend more time together. We went through photos and our parents' things, excavating memories and divvying up their possessions, the antique mirrors and intricate clocks that had populated our parents' and our own lives for so many years.

But still, after Mom's death it felt like I was moving through life with frayed edges. Throughout the day, I would reach for the phone to call her, to hear her voice. And every time the phone rang, my heart assumed it was her before my mind remembered she was gone. Allan was as devastated as I was. He had lost his dad unexpectedly just 10 days before my dad died, and losing his dad, then my dad, and now my mom—it all felt like too much.

Both of us were thinking of our own mortality. Allan was still managing his MS with vitamins and lots of rest, but there was always that fear that his symptoms might escalate. It had been 18 years since he had been diagnosed, and it was incredible that he was doing as well as he was, with only four to five major flares-ups each year. But lately, if he caught a cold, it lingered longer than usual, and that seemed to trigger a flare-up that led to dizziness, numbness, and pain in his limbs. And if he developed a fever, his symptoms only became worse. We were, it seemed, teetering on the edge of uncertainty.

I began to worry what would happen to the boys if Allan or I died. And what if Allan and I both died? What would happen to the boys then? I thought of my cousin Billy, who, after my aunt Frances died, lived on his own with some support services. He seemed fine, but I wondered how he felt. Did he feel abandoned?

Alie and Jamie would never be as independent as Billy had been, and I wondered who would take care of them when Allan and I were gone. Who would tuck them in each night? Who would fight for their happiness?

10

THE BOYS ALWAYS LOVED the ocean. Maybe it was the crashing of waves on sand. Maybe it was the way sunlight glinted off the water. I was never sure. But ever since that first visit to Florida when they were five, they loved going to the shore.

One day in late August when they were 15 years old, Randy and I took them out to Long Beach for the day. Randy had become so much more than a therapist and teacher and consultant; she had become a dear friend, and we all loved to spend time with her. Randy held Jamie's hand and I held Alie's as we raced into the chilly water and out, trying to beat the waves back to shore, over and over again. They watched the water splash around their ankles, smiles fixed on their tanned faces.

Randy and I laughed at how impossible it was to tire them out. Even with daily gym class at school and all the activities that Allan and I signed them up for—swimming, horseback riding, basketball— it was never enough to really exhaust them. At the beach, though, I was exhausted, so I finally told them it was time for lunch.

We had brought a picnic with us, so we rinsed the boys' hands and got them situated on the blanket with their sandwiches and apples. Then Randy and I sat down on our beach chairs and unwrapped our lunches. I took a deep breath, inhaling the salty air. It had been a difficult week at school for Alie, who had begun flailing his arms and hitting himself, his open hands slapping his body. I had been on edge all week, and I was up late every night updating his teachers on behaviors at home so we could develop a coordinated plan to address it. But today he seemed calmer, and I was grateful for that.

"Alie, Jamie, look at the birds!" Randy pointed up into the sky, to the seagulls that soared and dipped above the water. Both boys glanced up at the cawing birds and then down again to the sandwiches in their hands.

I hoped Alie was coming out of his latest rough patch. Since we first started him on medication at age 10, we had accepted that it was a necessity for him, and we had tried various medications and combinations of medications to help alleviate his anxiety and OCD. They had made a huge difference, but his OCD was still one of our biggest challenges.

As if on cue, Alie stood up, his sandwich abandoned on the sandy blanket so he could fix the cooler, which had shifted from its position when I opened it. He arranged it so that it was once again perfectly squared to the corner of the blanket, and then he began tapping on its blue lid.

I reached over and brushed off his sandwich, then patted the blanket. "Okay, Alie. It's okay. Sit down now. Time to eat."

Randy smiled, pulling her long curly dark hair over one shoulder. "I've been thinking about the boys' excess energy, Rob—especially Alie's—and I have an idea."

I turned to her. Randy knew the boys and their issues as well as anyone, and I knew if she had an idea, we'd try it. "What is it?"

Randy wiped her mouth with her napkin. "What if we could channel their energy and obsessiveness in a positive direction?" She paused. "Like running."

I could tell Randy was excited. She was a seven-time marathoner, and she often talked about the ways running had changed her life. In her mid-twenties she went from not running at all to running a 10K in six weeks. "You know I have some OCD tendencies, as well, and look what it's done for me!" She laughed then, and I laughed, too. It was true that like Alie, Randy liked to start and finish something. It was one of the reasons she'd fallen in love with running.

"The release of energy is so amazing. But also the focus and discipline." Randy's dark eyes almost seemed to sparkle. "Running has such a huge impact on overall wellness, but especially on reducing anxiety. And I've read it does great things for kids with disabilities."

When we were in our twenties, I went to aerobics a couple of times a week and Allan practiced martial arts and loved to scuba dive when we went on vacations, but neither of us had exercised regularly since the boys' diagnosis. When would we have had time? I loved the idea of getting the boys into running, though—anything to burn more of their energy. But I couldn't picture how it would work. Running seemed like such a solitary activity, and the boys would never be able to run alone. They were never more than three feet away from us or a teacher or caregiver. Not ever. How could they possibly run?

"I don't know," I said slowly. "How would that even work?"

I glanced at the boys. Jamie was leaning forward slightly, staring at the half-eaten sandwich in his hand, and he was vocalizing loudly: "Ahhh. Ahhhh. Mmmmmm. Eeeee. EeeEEE. Ahhhhh."

"It's okay, Jamie. Eat your sandwich." He took a bite and began to chew slowly. At this point, Jamie was still very compliant, still the easygoing one. Even if he hadn't been hungry, he would have eaten if I'd told him to eat.

Alie was eating fast, as he always did, taking a bite before he'd chewed and swallowed the previous one. His gaze was locked on the cooler, as if daring it to move even a centimeter from its designated spot. Sometimes I wish I could get inside his head, to feel what he felt. "Slow down, Alie," I said, putting my hand on his shoulder. "Don't forget to chew."

"There's a club here on Long Island called Rolling Thunder," Randy said. "They pair kids with disabilities with volunteer running guides. I know they have a number of kids on the spectrum on the team."

"But kids like Alie and Jamie?" There was a reason, of course, that autism was called a spectrum disorder. Some kids with an autism spectrum disorder (ASD) were extremely verbal and high functioning. They were able to communicate and understand directions. Some excelled in certain academic subjects or in music. They could drive cars and have girlfriends and go to college. They could get married some day. But Alie and Jamie were profoundly autistic. By this point I understood that on the spectrum, they were at the lowest end, having all of the characteristics of classic autism.

"I don't know," I said again. "Who could we trust to run with them?"

"The running coaches are supposed to be great," Randy said. "They pair them up based on speed and individual needs." She smiled. "I think the boys would love it. And I can run with them, too!"

Randy would do anything for the boys, and of course I would trust her to run with them; I'd trust her with anything. But still, running? One of our biggest fears had always been that the boys would run away or wander off and be hit by a car or end up drowning in a pond.

I glanced over at Jamie, who was still eating his sandwich. Alie was done with his lunch and had zeroed in on the plastic arm of my beach chair, his lean fingers beginning to tap, tap, tap.

"Linda knows the founder of Rolling Thunder. Ask her about it," Randy said.

Linda was the gym teacher at the Genesis School, and she certainly understood the boys' need for movement.

Randy stood up. "Alie," she said. Alie continued to tap.

I reached over and put my hand on top of his. "Quiet hands, Alie. It's okay." He stopped tapping. "Good job! Nice quiet hands."

Randy knelt down in front of him. "Alie, let's go run in the water!" Alie looked up and slipped his hand into Randy's and they were off.

I sat there with Jamie as he finished his lunch, which was a slow process because he kept getting distracted by the sand on the blanket. He'd brush it off only to have more sand appear—a losing battle. I reminded Jamie to eat again and watched Randy and Alie dash in and out of the surf. At one point they got caught by a wave and water splashed up their backs, but they didn't seem to mind. Randy let out a hoot of laughter, and I laughed as well, unable to resist her enthusiasm. The sun glinted off the water like a million shards of light.

———

A couple of weeks later I spoke to Linda and asked her what she thought of the boys running. "They'd do great," she said. "I told you how they've been running circles around the other kids in the gym. Especially Alie."

I nodded, remembering how she'd told me how fast Alie was getting. I imagined him as a cyclone, spinning through the warm air of the gymnasium, unstoppable.

"Can you tell me about Rolling Thunder?" I asked.

"Oh, they're fabulous!" she said. "I know the head coach. They've done wonders with so many kids with special needs."

"Really?" I asked, not yet believing that this might be a possibility for the boys.

Linda nodded. "And they run in mainstream races all over Long Island."

Mainstream races? I couldn't imagine Alie and Jamie running in a race with hundreds of other people, people without disabilities. But I felt the seed of something—hope?—begin to blossom inside me. And I knew that we were about to add running to the long list of other things we'd tried with them over the years, always searching for the thing that would make them the happiest.

"Okay," I said. "Let's see if they like it."

———

Linda put us in touch with Steve Cuomo, the founder of the Rolling Thunder Special Needs Program. Steve's voice on the phone was full of energy, almost boisterous. He told me that he had started Rolling Thunder in 1998 after he had taken his older son to participate in the Special Olympics and was told that his younger son, who did not have special needs, could not run with his brother. Steve explained that he wanted to create a team that was all about inclusion, a team where kids and adolescents with special needs could run with their typical peers and family members.

I was excited that this kind of team existed, but still I worried that Alie and Jamie with their profound needs would be unable to participate. But Steve wasn't about to take no for an answer. "We have a race coming up. Come and see what we're all about."

On the calendar, I wrote "Oyster Bay 5K" on Saturday, October 15. The race would kick off the annual Oyster Bay Festival, which drew crowds from all over Long Island. I remembered that Allan and I had gone there years ago, before the boys were born—a lifetime ago.

Alie and Jamie usually slept in on Saturday mornings, but that morning we got them up early so we could see a race in action. The drive from Great Neck was beautiful, and I thought of my mom as we passed the red and yellow trees, brilliant in the morning sun. She would have loved to be with us, heading to Oyster Bay for the festivities. I still felt the heaviness of grief when I thought about her, but also a surge of strength.

That summer when we were having trouble with Alie at school, his self-injurious behavior cropping up yet again, I would sit at my desk in our home office writing emails to the school team late at night and catch a glimpse of a note from her that I had taped to the wall: "Always with love to my treasured foursome." Then I'd turn to the photo that Mary had given me after Genesis opened all those years ago: "Nothing happens unless first a dream." Together, these messages gave me strength to keep going, keep searching for the right solutions for the boys, to always keep their well-being at the front of my mind. I should have also been thinking about my own well-being. I should have realized that I needed to take care of myself, as well. But it would still be years before I'd understand that.

On the way to Oyster Bay, Alie and Jamie stared out the car windows, their eyes darting back and forth like strobe lights. Were they memorizing the route? Or the pattern of fall colors? What was going on in their heads?

We had to park far from the finish line, but even with the long walk, we arrived just in time to see the first runners coming around the bend for the final stretch of the race. Thumping music filled my chest, and I could feel the thrill in the air. I held Alie's hand and Allan held Jamie's hand, and we found a spot at the curb to watch runner after runner cross the finish line. The Rolling Thunder runners wore green tank tops, and I was amazed by how many of them there were—some with noticeable disabilities but most of them not. Alie and Jamie were entranced, taking it all in, their eyes darting back and forth. Even as the last runners trickled in, the boys jumped up and down and bounced on the balls of their feet. It was as if they already knew they had found a home.

After the awards ceremony, Steve and a couple of other coaches welcomed us and we shook hands. "Say 'Hi,' Alie. Say 'Hi,' Jamie." Both boys murmured "Hi" and then looked away, their gazes returning to the trees, the sky, the cracks in the pavement, the movement of the crowd surrounding us.

"They look like runners," one of the coaches said. The others agreed: Alie and Jamie's long legs and slim builds were perfect for running. Steve told us a little more about the team and the training schedule, and as he spoke, he waved his arms in the direction of a group of Rolling Thunder runners. "There are endless possibilities for each one of my athletes. Our focus at Rolling Thunder is on their abilities, not their disabilities."

I loved Steve's attitude, but still, I was hesitant.

"Our athletes run at all different speeds and so do our volunteer coaches. We meet every Saturday morning at 9:00 AM at Sunken Meadow State Park."

Sunken Meadow was much farther out on Long Island than Great Neck; it hugged the banks of Smithtown Bay. Allan and I glanced at each other. I knew we were both thinking about the 45-minute drive there and back. Saturday and Sunday mornings were the only time that the boys slept late and the only time during the week that Allan and I were able to catch up on our own sleep. We'd have to get up by seven in order to get there in time.

"It may be hard for us to get out to Suffolk County that early in the morning. Are there any coaches closer to Great Neck who might be able to meet us closer to home this first time, just to see how the boys do?"

Steve smoothed his thick mustache and nodded, saying he thought he had just the coaches. "You can meet them in Eisenhower Park and see how the boys do. How about next Saturday?"

Eisenhower Park was only 20 minutes from our house, which felt much more manageable on a Saturday morning.

Allan nodded. "Okay, that sounds good. Thank you."

As we drove home, I felt nervous but also giddy. We had never considered having the boys participate in an integrated sport. Could it really be a possibility for Alie and Jamie?

I turned to look at Allan. "It sounds great, don't you think?"

Allan pursed his lips. "I don't know, Rob. We really don't know these people and they don't know the boys. The other runners...." Allan shrugged. "Steve said that a high percentage of the runners with

Rolling Thunder were on the autism spectrum, but it didn't appear that any of them had severe autism."

I agreed that what we faced with Alie and Jamie was completely different than what parents with high functioning kids with ASD faced. But still, it felt right to me. And the boys seemed so excited. "I know," I said. "But I think we should check it out." The least we could do was see how the boys did running with the coaches.

———

The following Saturday morning, Allan and I were up early, laying out breakfast for the boys in the kitchen. "Do you really think this is a good idea, Rob?" Allan said.

"I know," I said. It had been difficult for me to fall asleep the night before. What were we thinking? Were we really going to hand the boys off to strangers who didn't have any experience with kids with severe autism?

Since the boys had been diagnosed, we'd been protective, perhaps overly so, but who else would keep them safe?

"But they looked so happy at the race last weekend," Allan added, and I nodded.

"Wasn't that exciting?" I hadn't forgotten the sense of possibility I felt that day or the way the coaches had seemed to embrace Alie and Jamie—all of us. "I think we should try it. They might love it."

An hour later we pulled into the parking lot in the middle of Eisenhower Park. Shanthy and Mike, the coaches, were stretching nearby on the grass and waved to us as we helped the boys out of the car. Shanthy had an athletic build and long, dark hair pulled into a ponytail. Mike was fair-skinned and very thin. Alie and Jamie were fidgety as we approached them, and I worried that we'd made a mistake. *Were we really going to send them off with these strangers?*

But when we stopped in front of Shanthy and Mike, they both smiled warmly and extended their hands. "Wonderful to meet all of you," Shanthy said. "We've been looking forward to this."

I willed myself to relax. They were both warm and friendly—there was no reason to think they'd kidnap the boys or anything. But what if the boys ran away? Or hurt themselves? Alie had been so difficult to handle lately. What if he had a tantrum on the run and Mike and Shanthy couldn't calm him down?

"We're a little nervous," Allan said. "They've never done anything like this before."

Shanthy nodded. "We totally understand," she said. "It's a big step." She nodded at Mike. "But both of us have been volunteering with Rolling Thunder for a long time and we've worked with all sorts of kids. They're going to be fine."

"We'll stay close together," Mike added.

I wasn't sure how they would manage that, exactly, but it felt like time to let go, to loosen our grip a little. We told Shanthy and Mike to watch for specific behaviors, such as Alie's arm flapping and Jamie's loud vocalizing, which could mean they were upset about something. Shanthy and Mike nodded, not seeming at all nervous.

"Hi, Alie! Hi, Jamie! Are you ready to run?" Shanthy asked, and suddenly they were all off on a two-mile loop around the park.

The moment they ran out of sight, it felt as though I'd been punched in the stomach. Allan and I paced back and forth in the parking lot. Of course they'd only been gone a few minutes, but it felt like hours to both of us. We couldn't see them, and I kept thinking, *Please let them be okay. Why aren't they back yet?*

I started feeling lightheaded. I remembered when Jamie got lost at Disney World when the boys were six years old. We had stopped to ask directions and Allan briefly let go of Jamie's hand to pull a map from his back pocket. He let go of him for only a few seconds, but when he reached for Jamie's hand again, Jamie was gone. We screamed and ran around the crowded area of the park, yelling his name over and over again. Then I remembered the early training we'd done with

Jamie in our home program when we hid him around the house and taught him to come when we called his name. I steadied my voice and yelled, "Jamie, come here!" again and again as I walked through the crowds of people. I could feel my heart banging in my chest. I could hardly breathe. He had probably only been gone a few minutes, but it felt like hours. Suddenly he'd appeared, walking backward toward me while staring at some ride in the distance that had attracted his attention. I hugged him so tightly I could barely breathe. And I also sent up a prayer of gratitude for ABA and for the months of work we'd done with him in our home program.

If he came back when we called him at Disney World, surrounded by all those tantalizing distractions, certainly he would come when he was called now. He just wouldn't run off, would he? I was starting to panic. "Maybe this was a mistake," I said.

"I know," Allan said. His brow was furrowed, and I could tell he was just as nervous as I was.

Then suddenly, they came around the bend. Alie was out front, and he was flying. Then came Jamie and Mike and Shanthy. When the boys came to a stop in front of us, they both looked euphoric, smiling like we'd never seen before. Allan and I pulled them into tight hugs.

"They're naturals!" Mike said, breathing hard. "I've been coaching with the club for years and I've never seen anything like it, especially Alie. You should get them out as much as possible."

Shanthy nodded. "The only challenge is going to be to find a coach who is fast enough! We couldn't keep up!"

There was no question how the boys felt about running. They were beaming. The tight coil of worry in my chest gave way to something else: elation. It was the most amazing feeling to see them that happy. Allan put his arm around my shoulders and smiled down at me. "Let's sign them up," I said, and he nodded.

11

THE FOLLOWING SATURDAY morning I woke up early and began the process of getting the boys up and ready. I always woke Alie first because Jamie loved to sleep in as long as possible. I slipped quietly into Alie's room, though I don't know why I bothered being quiet; my presence always seemed to be enough to wake him. But he wouldn't move until I sat down on the edge of his bed and said, "Good morning, Alie."

"Moni," Alie responded softly.

"Do you want to go running today?"

His eyes flew open. "Yesss!" It was the clearest, most articulated "yes" he had said for a long time. Already I could see how running might become one of his biggest motivators.

Alie sat up and reached for his socks, and the morning routine was in motion.

Mornings were always complex for us. We had to be one step ahead of what we anticipated would happen with each of the boys based on recent behavioral problems and new obsessions. So we planned each moment, predicting what might happen, trying to thwart and redirect and keep everyone moving forward. If we didn't, we'd never make it out the door.

Alie quickly learned our wake-up routine and just as quickly developed compulsions around it, compelled to get each step right. He got up and walked with me to Jamie's room with Jamie's socks in his hand.

"Good morning, Jamie," I said.

Alie echoed me: "Moni, Jamie."

Jamie's head was deep under his blanket, but I heard a faint, "Good mornee, Alie."

Jamie emerged from his covers.

"Do you want to go running today?"

Another "Yes!"

Alie handed Jamie his socks.

I took both boys to the bathroom to brush their teeth and use the toilet. Because they had so many obsessive behaviors around clothes and their dressers, I always laid out their clothes for the next day downstairs in the den. If I left them to choose their own clothes, we'd end up in multiple compulsion loops: only a certain shirt on a certain day and only after 10 taps on the dresser, or something like that.

As soon as Alie brushed his teeth, he headed for the stairs. Alie had tripped down the stairs more than once and had also slammed into the wall on the landing. He was always rushing. Because of this, Allan was on guard at the bottom of the stairs to remind him to walk down slowly.

Alie didn't do "slow" without a lot of prompting, and we often had to make him go down the stairs several times before he could do it without charging them. But we didn't have time for that today, so we focused on having him chew and swallow each bite of his breakfast. Jamie, Alie's opposite, walked slowly down the stairs, dressed carefully, and chewed methodically, a distant smile on his face the whole time.

———

Allan and I had no idea what to expect of our first team practice with Rolling Thunder, but we were eager to try it. It was another beautiful fall morning, sunlight glinting through the trees as we drove the forty-five minutes to Sunken Meadow State Park. The boys sat in the backseat, their eyes darting back and forth as usual. This was a different route than we took last Saturday, so I wondered what they were thinking. "We're going to run with a team," I said, looking back at them. "Do you want to go running?"

Both boys glanced at me and mumbled "yes" again with dazed smiles.

"I hope they can take off right away," Allan said, and I nodded. The boys had never done well waiting, especially in new situations.

We pulled into the parking lot at Sunken Meadow and saw the team gathered on the grass, most of them wearing forest green Rolling Thunder windbreakers or Rolling Thunder tank tops over long-sleeve shirts. Parents congregated in small groups holding thermoses of coffee.

"Hi! Welcome!" Steve shouted, waving to us across the crowd.

The team was made up of boys and girls of all shapes and sizes with varying special needs. Most were teenagers like Alie and Jamie, but some of them couldn't have been more than eight or nine years old, and I felt a pang of regret, wishing that we had discovered how much they loved running sooner.

The runners were chattering away to each other or to the coaches, who were walking through the crowd, giving high fives. Some coaches were stretching and doing warm-ups with small groups of runners. Some of the kids would occasionally dash off and need to be called back and redirected. It was a little chaotic, but everyone seemed happy and excited to be there. It felt like one big family.

Allan and I held the boys' hands. Jamie was jumping and Alie was staring into the crowd, tapping his foot. As Allan had noticed at the Oyster Bay race, most of the athletes seemed to be higher functioning than Alie and Jamie, and I wondered if the severity of their autism would be a problem. Could they really run with a team?

"You're here!" Shanthy called, as she and Mike approached. "We're so happy you came!"

"We wouldn't miss it after last week," I said, smiling.

"They're ready," Allan said, nodding at the boys. "Or at least we hope so." He laughed.

Alie pulled on my arm and Jamie bounced, bounced, bounced.

Allan and I glanced at each other. I hoped the team would take off soon, before the bouncing and pulling turned into something else. Would they be able to handle this?

"Gather around," Steve yelled, and we moved forward with the boys. "Okay, everybody, listen up! As always we're going to be running in groups based on speed." Steve had been a star track and cross-country runner in high school, and he was serious about coaching and about treating the members of his team as runners rather than runners with disabilities. He began calling out names and pointing to the coaches who stood to one side. The kids began to split up and gather around the coaches to whom they were assigned.

Alie scraped his sneaker on the pavement and began to frenetically flap his hands. Uh oh.

"We're going to start off slow for the first loop," Steve yelled.

"The boys can come with us," Shanthy said, and she took Jamie's hand while Mike reached for Alie's.

"Have fun," Allan said.

Shanthy waved as they moved toward the cluster of runners.

"Okay people, let's go!" bellowed Steve.

And then they were off, heading uphill onto the dirt path and into the woods. Shanthy was running next to Jamie, Mike next to Alie. Alie had taken off fast and was pushing into the middle of the group of runners. How would they manage him? I felt anxiety ripple through me.

"Do you think they'll be okay?" Allan asked, his eyebrows raised.

"I'm sure they'll be fine," I said, and forced a smile.

Then Steve came over and shook our hands, smiling broadly. "We're so glad you're here!"

"We are, too," I said. "But we're a little nervous."

Steve shook his head, still smiling. "They're made to run! They're going to do great!"

It wasn't long before the pack of runners emerged from the trees on the other side of the park and headed across the meadow. Jamie was still running next to Shanthy, but Alie was up ahead, in the middle of the fast pack. He was carefully boxed in, with runners in front of him, on either side of him, and behind him. Mike was right there by his side. I'm sure he didn't understand why he was being held back, but I hoped he'd get used to it.

"They seem to have it under control," I said, relieved.

Allan slipped his hand into mine and gave it a squeeze.

The runners looped through the woods several more times, the slower groups falling back with each loop. When the run was over, the coaches helped the runners stretch in small groups. Each group was doing different stretches, which were constantly interrupted by the coaches' reminders to stay on task. All of that was understandable given the different levels of ages, abilities, and special needs, but it seemed a little hectic, and I could feel my urge to control the situation begin to percolate inside me.

But as I watched Alie and Jamie stretch alongside their peers, I realized that they both seemed fine—better than fine. They had ear-to-ear smiles. And because Alie and Jamie were so responsive to prompts, they did well stretching, bending when told to bend, pulling one arm then another across their chests when told to do that.

Allan and I stood to the side and watched, and I could feel myself begin to relax. Here were my sons, whom I never imagined would be able to run, and they were surrounded by other runners stretching on the grass. And I realized that this was only possible because of ABA. They learned how to learn, and that learning was generalizing to this new activity, an activity they seemed to love.

A short while later, when Allan and I handed the boys their sweat-shirts and got them into the car, a couple of other parents waved to us. "See you next week!" one shouted. We waved back, smiling.

We had been part of communities of autism parents before—when we gathered to launch Genesis and later, as Genesis parents. But so many of those group meetings were fraught with concerns: behaviors that couldn't be managed, services that we were all desperate to secure for our children. Rolling Thunder immediately felt like a community of people who understood what our lives were like, at least a little bit, but we were sharing a different goal: to have fun, to embrace the joy of running.

The whole way home, the boys were serene, smiling out the windows. And for the rest of the day, they were calmer than we'd seen them in ages, maybe ever.

———

The following week we again got up early and headed to Sunken Meadow. When Steve bellowed for the runners to gather around, Alie and Jamie just stood there by our sides. It was clear that they both needed one-to-one coaches for each practice. For the most part they were able to follow directions, but they couldn't navigate a crowd or fully grasp what was expected of them. And there was no telling whether they would just run off into the woods or not.

So each subsequent Saturday, they were assigned a specific coach. Shanthy most often ran with Jamie; she knew not to push him too hard to keep up the pace. If he felt pressured to run faster than was comfortable for him, he'd begin vocalizing loudly or reach out and touch her arm. Either Mike or Holly would run with Alie. Holly was a new volunteer coach for Rolling Thunder. She was a triathlete, tall and slender and very fast. She and Mike were the only coaches fast enough to catch up with Alie if he started sprinting away from the group. We had heard about another volunteer coach, Kevin, whom we were told was faster than any of the other coaches, but he hadn't been at any of the practices we'd attended so far.

A couple of times we also met Mike and Shanty separately at Eisenhower Park, which was closer to all of our houses. As much as we loved being a part of the team practices, it was sometimes easier to have the boys run with just Mike and Shanthy, especially if we'd had a hard week and all needed the extra sleep. Steve understood how difficult it was for us to get to Sunken Meadow each week, so he agreed that we could run separately when that was easier.

Mike joked that Alie only understood two words: go and stop. When he heard "go" he would run flat out, as fast as he could. When he heard "stop" he would come to a dead stop. Jamie, on the other hand, wasn't interested in speed at all; he just seemed to love to run. He almost skipped when he ran, and would just keep going. Jamie loved being with other people, and he loved swishy ponytails. When we practiced with the team, he would position himself behind a female runner with a swishy ponytail and follow her the whole way.

———

In late November, Shanthy told us about an upcoming race that she was planning to run with the team. It was the HoHoHo Holiday 5K in Bethpage, Long Island in mid-December. It was a mainstream race, and there would be over 1,000 people running it.

I wasn't sure if the boys were ready. Running with Mike and Shanthy at Eisenhower or Rolling Thunder at Sunken Meadow was one thing, but a race through the streets of Bethpage? What if one of the boys took off in the opposite direction and got hit by a car? How would Mike be able to pace Alie so he didn't sprint away from him?

On our way home from practice, I turned to Allan in the car. "What do you think? Should we sign them up?"

Allan shrugged. "They'd be running with Shanthy and Mike, who know them pretty well now."

"It would be so exciting, wouldn't it?" Aside from the annual gymnastics show when the boys were young, they had never participated in an athletic competition with their typical peers. But that was what Rolling Thunder was all about: inclusion. I glanced back at Alie and Jamie, who were still smiling from that morning's practice. Both were listening to their iPods, watching the play of light and shadows outside their windows.

"Let's do it," I said, and Allan reached over and squeezed my hand.

———

It was cold on December 17 when we woke early to get the boys ready for their first race. We got through our morning routine without a hitch and drove the 25 minutes to Bethpage. When we arrived, there were hundreds of runners milling around, stretching, and waiting in line for the porta potties, and I had a moment of panic. This was a completely different scenario than having them run in isolated Sunken Meadow Park. How would they handle running with all these people?

Allan and I moved through the crowds with the boys until we spotted a group of Rolling Thunder runners. Shanthy was handing out bibs, and she waved us over. We had dressed the boys in sweatpants, sweatshirts, and hats because it was only 33 degrees, but at the starting line we realized that we had over-dressed them. Most of the other runners only had long-sleeve shirts on. Some were even wearing shorts.

Allan and I pinned the race bibs onto the boys' sweatshirts and then we moved to the side and watched Shanthy and Mike lead them into the crowd of runners. Shanthy held Jamie's hand and Mike held on to Alie's hand. Alie and Jamie looked left and right, taking in the music and people, some of whom were decked out in Santa hats. They knew they were running; that was clear. They were both smiling broadly. But they didn't understand the significance of the moment.

They didn't understand that this was their very first race. They didn't understand that for the first time they would be running with a huge group of their typical peers. And neither they—nor Allan or I—could know that this was just the first of many races to come, that this was a new beginning for the boys, for all of us.

After the gun went off and all the runners filed past us, Allan and I moved to the other side of the course so we could see the boys coming around the corner toward the finish line. Luckily the route was a large rectangle, so we could see them both start and finish the race.

Allan and I pulled our hoods over our heads as we waited for the first runners to come around the bend. My hands were shaking, but I wasn't sure if it was from the cold or nerves. What if something went wrong? What if one of them became overwhelmed with the crowds?

Finally, Alie and Mike came around the corner, Alie's arms swinging down by his hips. Allan and I screamed his name into the cold air. "Go, Alie! Go!" Mike had been able to keep him from sprinting, and they finished in 27:45. He did it!

We ran over to the finish line to get to him. He was breathing heavily and sweating. It was clear that sweatshirts and woolen hats were not ideal running attire. But that didn't seem to faze Alie; he was radiant.

We moved with Alie and Mike back to the side of the road so we could see Jamie and Shanthy come in, and a few minutes later they appeared. Jamie loped alongside Shanthy, his eyes intent on the finish line, which they crossed at 31:24. "Go, Jamie! Go!" We ran over and hugged Jamie and gave him high fives. "Did you have fun, Jamie?"

"Yes," he said simply, smiling.

Allan and I thanked Shanthy and Mike.

"They did great!" Shanthy said.

Then Allan and I gave each other a big hug. Neither of us could believe that our sons had finished their first race, a race with a thousand runners who, unlike them, didn't have severe disabilities. I wished my parents had been alive to see it. They would have been so proud.

12

SATURDAY MORNING RUNS became our new routine, and Alie soon calibrated his internal clock and his obsessive-compulsive behaviors accordingly. On Friday evenings after dinner, he would find the cooler in the pantry and set it on the kitchen floor. He would then fill it with bottles of water and Gatorade. Then he'd go get his and Jamie's running shoes from the den and arrange them on the floor in a crescent. The shoes had to be spaced just right, the laces pulled taut to the sides of each shoe. He also became obsessed with his running clothes. If he saw his running clothes in the laundry basket, he would immediately want to put them away in the closet or drawer. Initially, we thought it was cute that he wanted to help with chores. But then his obsession transferred to any clothes that he thought were out of place around the house. He would pull dirty clothes from the hamper, fold them, and put them away. He would race down to the basement and find his running clothes hanging on the line to dry, and he would bring them upstairs, soaking wet, and try to press the sopping mess into his drawer.

Before breakfast, Alie retrieved his orange Nike running bag from the pantry and would arrange it on the chair next to him so that its straps would be hidden under the bag. As he ate, he'd stare at it and make sure it didn't shift at all. This bag symbolized running. Even if we didn't need it, Alie insisted it come with us. We packed it with extra shirts, gloves, hats, and socks for the boys, and Alie would inspect the contents before each run. Everything related to running was now sacred.

Jamie was clearly excited about running as well, but like so many things, Jamie embraced our new routine joyfully rather than obsessively. Alie tried to rush him through dressing and cereal, waiting at the door to put Jamie's hat on for him, but luckily Jamie didn't seem to mind. After practice, Jamie would sit in the backseat of the car, smiling and humming one of his favorite songs, carefree and relaxed. Years later, it would be hard to imagine Jamie like that, so easygoing. But when the boys were 15, he was, and he would go along with just about anything.

We began to get to know some of the coaches and the other athletes and their families, and they were all warm and accepting. As special needs parents, there existed among us a sense of understanding and camaraderie. None of us needed to explain away behaviors or differences.

Some of the parents were also coaches and they ran alongside their children. Neither Allan nor I had ever been runners, so it didn't even cross my mind to run with Alie and Jamie. And of course we wouldn't have been fast enough to run with Alie anyway. So Allan and I stood at the edge of the meadow and watched the boys loop into and out of the woods with the team.

At the beginning of February, Randy convinced us to register the boys for the Snowflake 4 Mile Run in Long Beach, which she and Joanne were planning on running. Four miles was a little farther than the boys had been running, so I was hesitant, but Randy convinced me it would be fine. And I loved the idea of the boys running with Randy and Joanne, who had been through so much with us. So we signed them up and decided that Randy and Mike would run with Alie and Shanthy and Joanne would run with Jamie.

A frigid wind was coming off the ocean when we got out of the car in Long Beach, so I was grateful when we stepped into the gym at the school, where we were picking up the boys' bibs and meeting Joanne, Randy, Shanthy, and Mike.

Randy and Joanne were beaming, both dressed in long shirts, tights, and thin hats. Like Randy, Joanne was a longtime runner, and I knew she was just as excited as Randy to be running with the boys.

"Hi Alie! Hi Jamie!" They both gave the boys big hugs.

The boys jumped up and down, smiling. We pinned the race bibs onto their long-sleeve shirts and headed back out into the freezing air.

Randy rubbed her hands together, smiling. "Isn't this amazing?"

"I know," I said. It was hard to believe that it had been less than six months since she suggested we get the boys running, and now they were moving toward the starting line of their second mainstream race.

At the starting line, Randy and Mike took Alie and walked toward the front, and Joanne and Shanthy moved into the center of the pack with Jamie. When the gun sounded, off they went.

It was an out-and-back race that went down the road and came back on the boardwalk. They had both done so well in the HoHoHo race, so we shouldn't have been worried, but we knew anything could happen. But we also knew how much the boys loved to run. They would be fine, probably better than fine.

We paced back and forth in the cold wind, trying to stay warm.

"It's freezing!" Allan said.

"I know!" I said, but we were both smiling.

The runners began to come in, and finally we saw Alie and Randy and Mike, racing toward us down the boardwalk. Randy was reaching for Alie's shirt. Mike was just behind them. Randy looked strained. "I hope she's okay," I said to Allan.

A few minutes later when they made their way toward us on the sideline, Randy was shaking her head. "He's crazy fast! So focused, no behaviors. He was amazing!"

"He only knows one speed—fast!" Mike laughed.

"I kept having to tell him to slow down!" Randy said, still shaking her head.

Allan and I hugged Alie. "Great job, Alie!" And then Allan helped him slip on his jacket. Alie seemed utterly calm, euphoric.

"His form isn't great, though," said Randy.

I nodded. It was true that Alie ran with his arms down, swinging like pendulums.

She laughed. "Think what he could do if he was running more efficiently!"

A minute later, Jamie appeared with Joanne and Shanthy running on either side of him. They were all grinning, their faces flushed. We all yelled, "Go, Jamie!"

Joanne was laughing moments later when they found us. "He's incredible!" she said. "So happy."

We hugged Jamie and helped him pull his sweatshirt over his head.

Shanthy nodded. "He could have run another four miles."

"Did you have fun, Jamie?" Allan asked.

"Yessss," he said, still smiling.

Later, I felt awful when I found out that Randy had developed shin splints as the result of sprinting after Alie down the boardwalk. We realized we had to either slow him down or find him a faster coach.

That's when we met Kevin McDermott, the fast Rolling Thunder coach about whom we'd heard. Kevin had been volunteering for Rolling Thunder for almost a year, but he wasn't at every practice and neither were we, so our paths didn't cross until later that month when we showed up one Saturday morning and he was the coach assigned to Alie.

Sometimes people come into our lives and later we can't imagine what we'd do without them. Kevin was—is—just such a person.

That morning when we arrived at Sunken Meadow, Steve shook our hands. "I'm glad you're here! You can finally meet Kevin. He'll be running with Alie today."

Steve walked us all over to where Kevin was standing with a group of the fastest Rolling Thunder athletes. "Kevin! I want you to meet the Schneiders."

Allan and I introduced ourselves and Alie and Jamie. "Hello!" he said, smiling warmly, shaking our hands. "I've heard a lot about all of you." Kevin had the chiseled face of a serious runner.

We explained that Jamie was doing well running with Shanthy's group but that Alie was unpredictable, sometimes staying with the faster group and other times sprinting out ahead of them. Kevin nodded as we talked to him about Alie's needs and lack of ability to communicate.

I usually felt nervous when Alie was running with a new coach at practice, but Kevin seemed so calm and confident. He was tall and lean and had the look of an elite runner. Years later, he'd laugh and say, "Ha! I had no idea what I was getting into!"

But off Alie went with him and a small group of the fastest Rolling Thunder runners. We watched them loop through the meadow and into the forest again and again, and Alie seemed to be doing well, staying with the group.

After that practice, I asked Kevin how it went.

"He's definitely fast," he said, smiling. "Our biggest issue is going to be pacing, especially that first mile or two." Kevin told us how Alie had taken off fast and gotten away from the group. "Luckily, the other boys are fast, too, so I sent one of them after Alie to tell him to stop. When we got Alie back with the group, we encircled him and ran like that." He shook his head. "But he kept breaking free."

"We call him 'One Speed Only,'" I said, and Kevin laughed.

"I'd love to see what he can do," said Kevin. We'd soon learn that's how Kevin was: curious, supportive, competitive. Years later, he'd still be doing just that: seeing what Alie could do, pushing him to run times indicative of his ability.

We learned that Kevin had started running in Thailand, where he and his wife, Leslie, had lived and taught for a number of years while they were serving as missionaries. On a whim, he began running with a fellow teacher who was training for the Bangkok Marathon, and he ended up falling in love with it.

Whenever Kevin was at practice, Alie was assigned to run with him, but Kevin was juggling a lot and couldn't make it to all of the practices. He and Leslie had returned to the States from Thailand in 2004 after Kevin's sister and her husband died tragically within a few months of each other. They moved back to Long Island to raise their teenage nieces. Now they also had a young daughter, Mercy, whom they adopted from Thailand in 2005. He and Leslie had their hands full, but somehow he still found time to make it to most practices that spring, and we were grateful.

———

It felt like a time of renewed hope. I'd spent the previous year dealing with my mom and dad's affairs, which was exhausting and seemed endless. But by the beginning of 2006, everything was pretty much in order. Their Florida condo and their East Meadow house had finally been sold, and I was ready to shake off the shroud of grief that had been clinging to me since my mom's death.

Both of the boys' behaviors were erratic, up and down as they had always been, but since they had started running, they both seemed happier. On running days, their anxious energy was being directed in a positive way and they had fewer problematic behaviors. Running was somehow different from all the other activities they had participated in over the years. It was something special that more and more felt like a new start.

When you have an older child with severe autism, you have already spent years and years leaping over and around so many roadblocks that it's easy to stop thinking about the future in a positive way. You

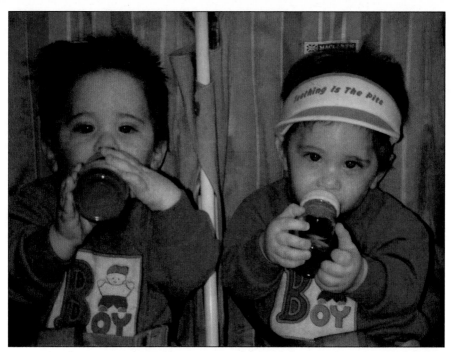

Jamie (left) and Alex (right) at one year old (1991).

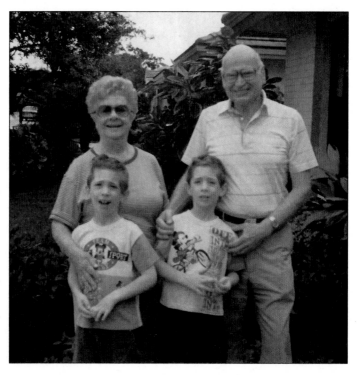

Alex (left) and Jamie (right) at five years old with their grandparents, Frances and Ingram, in Florida (April 1996).

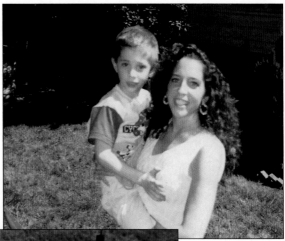

Alex and Ruth at Alex and Jamie's sixth birthday party (1996).

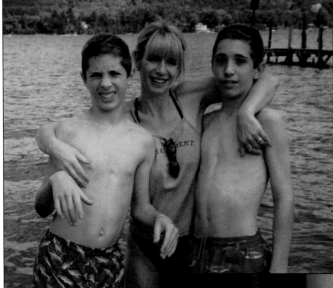

Jamie (left), Robyn, and Alex (right) at 12 years old on a summer vacation in upstate New York (2002).

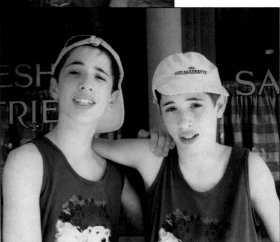

Alex (left) and Jamie (right) at 13 years old at Walt Disney World, Orlando, Florida (2003).

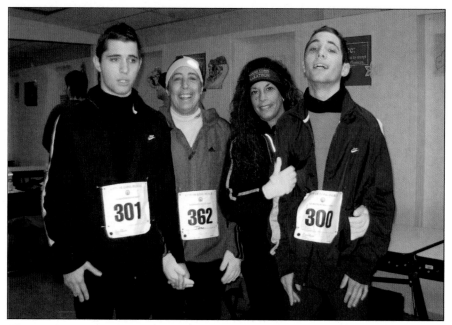

From left to right: Jamie, Joanne, Randy, and Alex at 17 years old at the 4 Mile Snowflake Run, Long Beach, New York (2007).

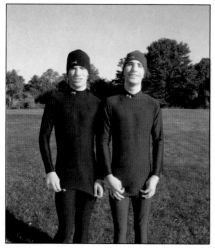

Jamie (left) and Alex (right) at 17 years old at Bethpage State Park, New York (2007).

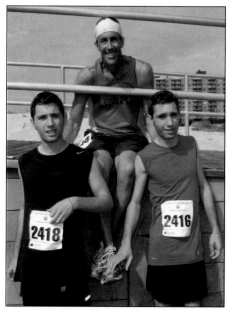

From left to right: Jamie, Kevin, and Alex at 19 years old at the Robert McAvoy Labor Day 5 Mile Run, Long Beach, New York (2009).

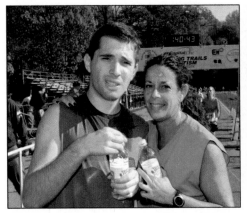

Jamie at 19 years old, and Randy, at the Blazing Trails 4-Autism Four Mile Run, Great Neck, New York (2009).

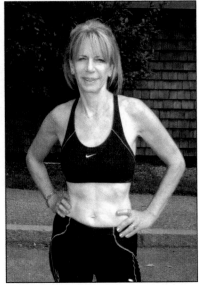

Robyn on a family vacation in New Hampshire.

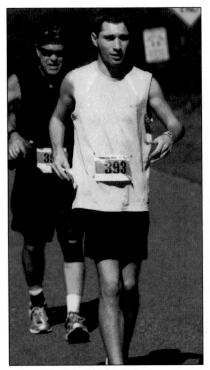

Allan and Jamie at 20 years old at the Hamptons Marathon (2010).

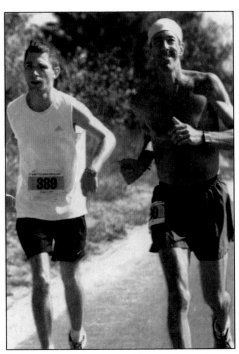

Alex at 20 years old and Kevin at the Hamptons Marathon (2010).

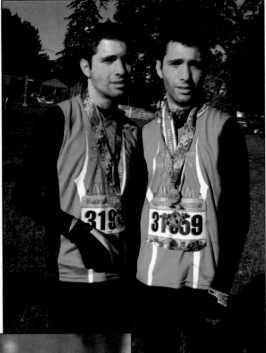

Jamie (left) and Alex (right) at 21 years old at the Marine Corp Marathon (in Washington, DC, 2011).

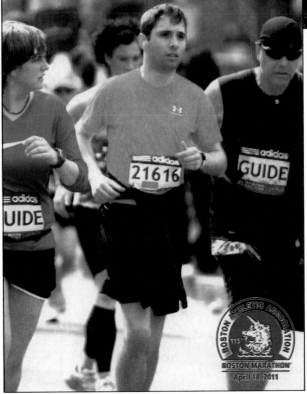

Katie, Jamie at 21 years old, and Allan at the Boston Marathon (2011).

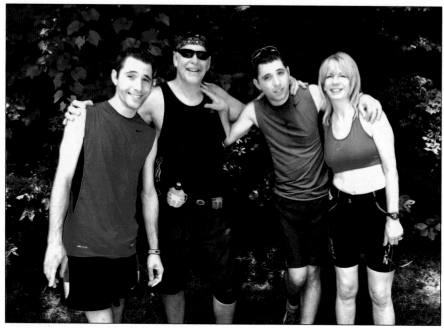

Alex and Jamie at 22 years old, Allan, and Robyn on a family vacation in Connecticut (2012).

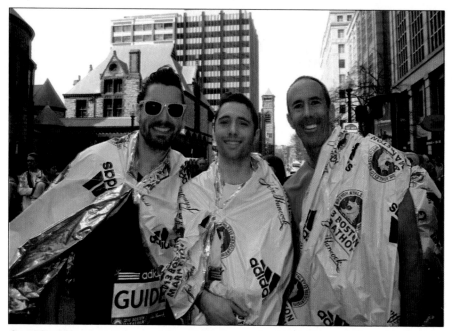

Stephen, Alex at 23 years old, and Kevin at the 2013 Boston Marathon before the bombs were detonated.

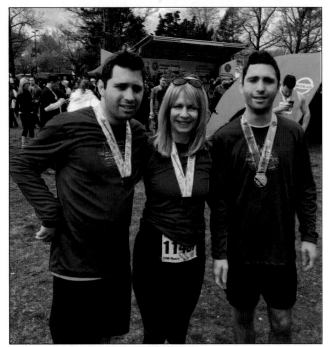

Jamie, Robyn, and Alex at 23 years old at the Long Island Festival of Races, East Meadow, New York (2014).

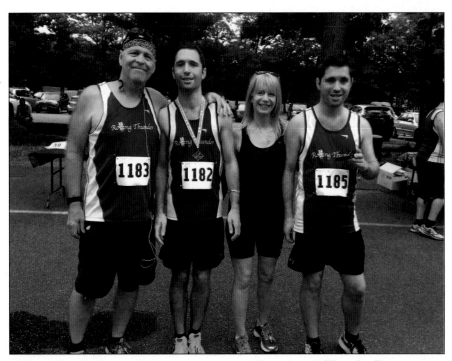

Allan, Alex, Robyn, and Jamie at 24 years old at the 5K Thunder Run, Hauppauge, New York (2014).

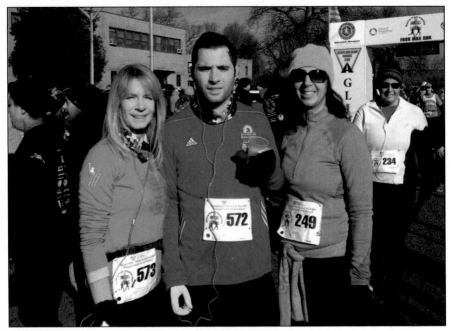

Robyn, Jamie at 24 years old, and Shanthy at the Blazing Trails 4–Autism Run (2014).

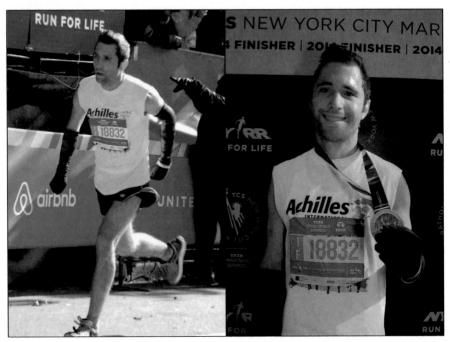

Alex at 24 years old, approaching the finish line (left) and with finisher's medal (right) at the TCS New York City Marathon (2014).

know that as soon as you've dodged one roadblock, another will pop up. The future is more daunting than it is filled with promise. But Rolling Thunder and the boys' running cracked something open in us. It made us consider once again our sons' capabilities, their talents. We could sense their potential. Maybe they could sense it, too.

Because I had finally finalized my parents' affairs, I also had time to consider working again. I realized I didn't want to return to management, though. What I really wanted to do was somehow make a positive impact on families struggling with autism. I felt a pull to do more, to make a difference not only in my sons' lives but also in the lives of all families living with autism. So one day while I was talking to Joanne, I asked her whether Eden II had ever thought of creating a government relations position. In my previous job, one of my responsibilities was to seek out and secure grants for various programs to help vulnerable people and families in need. Because Eden was so well-established and respected and because there was growing awareness and concern over increased rates of autism, I knew funding could be made available for the Eden II schools if there was someone dedicated to pursuing it.

"We've had wonderful support on Staten Island for years and now on Long Island," Joanne said. "But I agree that there's potential for more services if we had the funds. Put together a proposal and I'll discuss it with the executive team."

That's how Joanne was—she made things happen. When the board and executive team approved adding a legislative coordinator position to Eden's staff, I applied for it. It had benefits, which we still needed. But it was part-time, so I would still have time with the boys and Allan. And it was exactly the kind of job I hoped for: I would be working to secure funding for projects and services that would not only make a difference in Alie and Jamie's lives but in the lives of others affected by ASD.

I was hired that spring, and it was the perfect fit. I loved working with Eden's executive team on funding initiatives that would ensure that the school would be around for years to come. I lobbied state senators and assembly members and raised money for video training programs, after-school programs, teacher and staff development, and crisis and respite care. The paperwork and contract management with various state departments was intense, but I didn't mind; I was helping to connect kids with autism and their families with needed services and supports.

———

That same spring, Linda, the physical education teacher at Genesis who first connected us with Rolling Thunder, signed the boys up for the 1500 meter race at the New York–Long Island Region's 35th Annual Special Olympics Spring Games. The boys had participated in events such as ball tossing and balance and jumping when they were younger, but we hadn't attended in years.

That year it was being hosted at Great Neck South High School, which would have been Alie and Jamie's high school had they not had such severe autism. When the boys were young and I drove by the high school it seemed like a beacon of hope: they would be cured of autism and end up as typical sophomores, juniors, seniors. When I realized that they would not only never be cured but that they also would never be mainstreamed, I hated driving by the school. It became of symbol of everything we'd lost. But now that running had come unexpectedly into our lives and had given us a renewed sense of potential, driving by South no longer bothered me. It seemed like the perfect place to highlight the boys' new passion.

Allan and I were a little nervous, as always. They expected a crowd of more than 4,000 people, and the boys would not only be running on the track for the first time, they'd be running without coaches. What if they ran off the track and into the crowd?

Allan was in Minnesota visiting his mother, which made me even more anxious. I couldn't handle the boys in a crowd on my own if one of them had a tantrum or ran off. Luckily, two of our home therapists, Debbie and Cathy, agreed to accompany me so we could position ourselves around the edges of the track and catch them (hopefully) if they got away.

The school campus is beautiful—full of rolling hills and winding paths—and the day of the Special Olympics was gorgeous. The boys participated in ball tossing first and enjoyed it, just as they had when they were young. Then Debbie and Cathy and I led them to the track, where Linda, who helped coordinate the event, was waiting for us. They had never run on a track, but as soon as they saw it they began jumping and smiling. They knew they'd get to run.

The bleachers were packed with cheering people. There were four other teenage boys competing in the 1500 meter. They were talking to one another as they stretched and warmed up. They were probably on the spectrum, as well, but as I walked the boys to their starting positions, I was struck by how severe Alie's and Jamie's autism was in comparison. Though they could answer simple questions, they couldn't have a conversation. They could not tell me what they did during school, what they ate for lunch, or how they felt about any of it. Was it even right for me to let them compete against these boys?

Linda lined up Alie in the first position and Jamie next to him, then directed the other boys to their lanes. I just wanted the boys to have fun, as they had tossing the ball back and forth. And of course, I wanted them to stay on the track. But when the gun went off, Alie and Jamie seemed to understand that this was a race. They sprinted around that first bend and just kept going. The crowd cheered. I screamed at the top of my lungs. "Go Alie! Go Jamie! Run fast! Go!"

I got so caught up in the moment that I didn't even realize that the boys had pulled away from the other runners. When they passed me, Alie was out front, Jamie not far behind him. I stood at my post on the side of the track, admiration and joy and disbelief all mixed together as I watched them hurtle around the track again and again.

Alie finished in first place in 6:05 and Jamie in second place in 6:23. More than overjoyed, I was shocked. Debbie and Cathy and I were all screaming and hugging the boys, unable to believe that they not only ran on a track, alone, but that they came in first and second places. I wished Allan had been there. I couldn't wait to tell him about it.

When the boys climbed onto the podium that was set up on the grass in the center of the track, I felt my eyes burn. Alie stood on the top middle position, Jamie on the right, the teenager who took third place on the left. As a medal was slipped over each of their heads, I snapped photo after photo—not that I would ever need them to remind me of that day. I would never forget my sons' proud smiles or how far they had come as runners in such a short time.

13

RUNNING WAS CLEARLY SOMETHING the boys not only loved but were really good at, so we realized it was time to invest in real running gear and proper running shoes. Up to this point, they had been running in regular sneakers, everyday t-shirts, sweats, and nylon shorts. A couple of Rolling Thunder coaches recommended we take them to Runner's Edge, a store in Farmingdale near Bethpage State Park that offered discounts to Rolling Thunder athletes.

So after a Saturday practice, we drove to Farmingdale and parked on Main Street in front of Runner's Edge, which was a small store, its walls lined with colorful running shoes and, in the back, racks of spandex and dry-fit clothes. When we walked through the door we were greeted by a friendly young man.

"Hi," I said, smiling. "We need shoes for our sons." I motioned to Alie and Jamie, who stood between Allan and me. Jamie bounced, bounced, bounced on the soles of his feet.

"The boys have autism," Allan said. "So they might not be too cooperative."

Alie started pulling on my arm to leave, already getting restless.

"No problem," the salesman said. Then he turned to Alie and Jamie. "And who do we have here?"

"This is Alie," Allan said, placing one hand on Alie's shoulder. "And this is Jamie." He placed his other hand on Jamie's shoulder.

"Okay, Alie and Jamie," he said, smiling at the boys. "Let's measure your feet and find the right shoes for you."

Sometimes when we tell a stranger that Alie and Jamie have autism, it seems as though they stop seeing the boys as real people. They may glance at them out of curiosity, but they don't speak directly to them. They don't hold out their hand for them to shake. I know that sometimes people just don't know how to act around my sons; perhaps they're worried that they'll do or say the wrong thing. And certainly it's true that the boys are easily agitated. But I'm always grateful when we meet someone who seems to really see them.

Maybe this man knew other people with disabilities. Maybe he'd helped other Rolling Thunder athletes with special needs who had shopped at the store. Regardless, I was relieved that he not only did not seem frazzled by the boys; he welcomed us.

He spent time looking at Alie and Jamie's feet, then pulled down a few different brands he thought might work. "They're all good shoes."

"I like the look of these," I said, pointing to the Sauconys.

The salesman nodded and said he'd check for their size. He disappeared for a moment and returned with a stack of boxes.

We had the boys each try on a pair, and the salesman pressed on their toes to make sure they fit properly. "Let's test these out," he said, and we all walked to the hallway near the back of the store. We told the boys to run back and forth, and they happily complied, though they probably wondered what the heck was going on. They seemed to like the shoes, though, so we bought two pairs: one in gray and orange for Jamie and the other in gray and blue for Alie, so we could tell them apart.

Later that week, I also went shopping and bought them running shorts and dry-fit t-shirts, tank tops, and long sleeves. The next time we went running, I couldn't believe how handsome they were; they now looked like real runners.

———

Alie and Jamie ran with the team on Saturday mornings all that spring and into the summer. Both boys were getting faster, shaving a couple of minutes off their 5K times, and several coaches, including Kevin, mentioned how great it would be if we could get them out running more than once a week.

Although Rolling Thunder had Tuesday and Thursday night practices as well as Saturdays, it was difficult for us to make the weeknight practices. Sunken Meadow was just too far from our house, especially when our late afternoons and evenings were filled with therapy and dinner and our lengthy bedtime routine, which included Allan and me showering the boys and getting them ready for bed, a two-hour process.

Then, in July, Joanne had a brilliant idea. Randy and the boys and I had met Joanne in Long Beach to spend the day by the ocean. As we sat on our beach chairs watching the waves, I told them what the coaches had said about getting the boys to run more and they both agreed. "Think what they could do!" Randy said.

"Not to mention the impact it could have on their behaviors," Joanne added, taking a sip of her water.

She was right. The days that the boys ran, they came home calmer, were less agitated all afternoon, and fell asleep easily. I would love to spread that out over the whole week. "That would be great," I said, opening a bottle of water for Jamie and handing it to him. "But it's a challenge because we can't make it to the evening practices, and if Kevin can't make it to practice, Alie has to skip his weekly run altogether because there aren't really any other coaches who can run fast enough to catch him if he gets away."

Joanne laughed. "He was running like a lunatic in the Snowflake race. Randy, do you remember?"

"How could I forget?" Randy said, patting Alie's hand. "He would sprint, then slow down, then sprint all out again. He was pounding down the boardwalk, scaring the pants off of everyone ahead of him."

"They just love it, though," I said, smiling at the boys, who were both staring out at the waves, Jamie slowly eating his apple and Alie tapping tapping tapping on the arm of his beach chair.

Joanne looked up at me, shielding her eyes from the sun with her hand. "I've got an idea."

"What?" I asked, pulling my hair away from my neck.

"Why don't you and Alie follow me to my garage? Let's see how he does if I bike alongside him."

"I don't know, Joanne. Biking?" I said, wary. "What if he runs into you and knocks you over? Or what if he starts to sprint and gets away from you?" I pictured Alie taking off and heading straight across the sandy beach and into the waves.

But Joanne always had great suggestions, so even as I imagined one disaster then another, I knew I'd agree to give it a try.

Joanne was already standing, brushing sand from her shorts. "I wouldn't do this if I wasn't confident that Alie would listen to me."

Joanne was right. She had excellent stimulus control over Alie; he listened to her like a soldier. If anyone could do this, it would be her.

"Okay," I said. "Let's see how he does."

"I'll keep Jamie here with me," said Randy, holding out her hand to Jamie. "Come on, Jamie, let's go jump in the waves."

I held my hand out to Alie. "Do you want to go running, Alie?"

He looked up at me, smiling. "Yesss."

Luckily, I had their running shoes in my car, which was parked across from the beach. Alie changed into his shoes as Joanne got her bike from her garage and walked it back to the boardwalk.

Even though we'd never done this before—it would never have occurred to me—Alie seemed to understand. He watched Joanne intently as she got on her bike and positioned herself on the boardwalk.

"Okay Alie," she said. "Do you want to run?"

"Yessss."

"Okay then. We're going to run now, but you have to stay with me. If I say 'stop' you stop. Okay, Alie?"

"Yessss."

Then they were off down the boardwalk. It was a Saturday in late July, so the boardwalk was crowded, but luckily it had a designated path for bikes. Joanne had Alie stay to her right, close to the line separating the bikers from the pedestrians. Soon they were out of sight, and I took a deep breath. *I'm sure they're fine.* But I kept imagining collisions involving multiple pedestrians. Now that he'd experienced the "runner's high" he seemed to want to sprint all out whenever he had the chance. He had tasted freedom.

I turned toward the beach, which was dotted with bright yellow and blue and rainbow umbrellas. I squinted in the bright sun and scanned the shoreline until I spotted Jamie's pale blue t-shirt and Randy's orange t-shirt and dark hair. They were running into the surf, jumping over waves, and I could tell they were having fun. I watched them for a few minutes, grateful for the ocean breeze and for my friends, who had done so much for the boys.

Then I turned around and waited for Joanne and Alie, trying not to let anxiety take hold of me. I glanced at my watch. They had been gone for almost fifteen minutes. Again an image of mangled collision flashed through my mind. This was a mistake. But suddenly Joanne and Alie appeared: Alie pounding toward me on the boardwalk, his arms swinging low and fast, Joanne beside him pedaling away.

I smiled. They did it! It worked! No catastrophes.

When Joanne and Alie came to a stop in front of me, they were both breathing hard but smiling.

"I knew he'd be able to do it," Joanne said, clearly pleased with the results of all their ABA training. "Alie and Jamie learned how to learn. Sure, they have difficult behaviors, but when they're not going through a rough time, they're compliant." She spoke the way she always had, straightforward and encouraging. "He can do this! You can do this with him!"

———

I hadn't been on a bike in probably 20 years. Before Allan and I were married, we tried riding through Great Neck a few times, but the town is so hilly that we ended up walking our bikes almost half the time. We laughed and decided it would make more sense to ditch the bikes and just go for walks. We didn't even own bikes anymore. But clearly we needed them. If Alie could do this, then certainly Jamie would be able to, as well. And if we could ride alongside them, we could make sure they ran more than once a week.

Allan and I bought bikes later that week, and from then on, if Kevin wasn't going to be at practice, Jamie could run with Shanthy, and Allan or I could bike with Alie as he ran.

But it turned out that biking alongside Alie was hit or miss. Some days he was great and would respond if we told him to slow down. Other days he'd sprint out way ahead, and we'd have to pedal hard to catch him. I had good stimulus control over Alie, so for the most part, he stayed with me and listened when I told him to slow down, but still, it was nerve-wracking. I peddled as fast as I could, but it wasn't fast enough for Alie. And anytime we got to a hill, I had to slow down even more, and Alie would charge up the hill ahead of me.

But even though it wasn't easy to bike with Alie, I loved watching him run. Usually I only saw him before and after runs, but seeing him in action was entirely different. It was as if the motion of his feet hitting the pavement settled him into an alternate state. Any disruptive behaviors that existed outside of running ceased. He was totally calm, totally Zen. Had I been able to keep up, he would have run and run and run, silent and focused.

———

I would have kept biking with Alie on days Kevin couldn't make practice, but that fall I developed vertigo. I'm not sure what brought it on, but one night I woke up with the world reeling. I was terrified. "Allan," I said, reaching for him in bed. "Everything is spinning. I can't sit up!"

Allan turned on the light.

"Call Dr. Gupta," I said, feeling as if I'd throw up.

"Now? Its 3:00 in the morning!"

"Yes. Please. Call him." I had a wonderful relationship with my internist, Dr. Gupta, who had also been my mom's doctor for years and years and had been so kind to me after her death.

Allan dialed Dr. Gupta's number and then handed me the phone. I left a message and he called me back immediately. He told me not to worry, that I probably had benign paroxysmal positional vertigo (BPPV). There are crystals in our inner ears that can be dislodged and fall into the ear canal, which then becomes sensitive to head position changes. Even the slightest movements can cause dizziness. He told me that I could try physical therapy but that it would probably just have to run its course. He recommended the anti-nausea medication Bonine to relieve the dizziness.

But "dizziness" didn't begin to describe my vertigo. The room began to spin if I didn't keep my head perfectly straight when I bent down or walked. I had a hard time sleeping at night because if I shifted, I was sent into orbit, our bedroom a planet off its axis. I couldn't drive, and I felt nauseated if I turned my head quickly or stood up too fast. I was living in slow motion.

I had always been healthy, and I wasn't used to thinking about how I moved or didn't move my body. I think the boys sensed that something was wrong, because they were unusually quiet around me. Alie didn't pull on my arm the way he sometimes did, and Jamie didn't jump around me as much as usual. I felt badly that I couldn't hug them or play around as much, but they seemed to understand.

Luckily a few of our wonderful home therapists, particularly Joe and Debbie, stepped in to work extra hours. Joe had been with us for a couple of years, and both boys delighted in him, but especially Alie. Joe had a spunky energy that both excited and somehow calmed Alie. It was such a relief to know that the boys were in good hands as I struggled to keep my balance.

During those weeks of vertigo, it was impossible to even consider riding a bike, so Allan took over biking with Alie. But because Allan hadn't been as involved in the boys' therapy and behavior plans, he didn't have as much stimulus control over Alie as I did. So Alie would test him. If Allan told him to slow down, Alie would ease up for a minute and then begin sprinting again. They would dodge people, weaving on and off the path the whole way. Alie was running, yes, but it clearly wasn't ideal for either of them.

Years later, Kevin would wonder whether Alie's tendency to sprint full speed had to do with the fact that he didn't know when he'd be able to run again. Would it be once a week or twice? If he showed up to practice not having run in a week or more, and without knowing when he'd be running again, he certainly wasn't going to waste the opportunity to let it all out. So he did. He let it all out.

My vertigo finally subsided after about six weeks, and it was such a relief to feel like myself—or almost myself—again. I realized that though I had been living with the effects of Allan's MS for 20 years, I had always taken *my* health for granted, and I could no longer do that.

I started seeing a naturopath whom Allan had seen interviewed on the news. At first I was skeptical, but my dad and Allan had always been huge believers in naturopathic medicine, so I agreed to give it a try. And I ended up loving Dr. Stills; she was delightful and had an impressive knowledge of how to best integrate conventional medicine with ancient Eastern therapeutics. It just felt right to me. I started taking supplements to boost my immune system, and I changed my diet to include more vegetables and fruit, eliminating everything with artificial coloring or flavoring. I began to prepare a healthy smoothie each morning with almond butter, greens, vanilla protein, strawberries, and bananas. She also encouraged me to carve out time for myself, and I agreed I'd try, but since the boys' diagnosis, I'd struggled with that. Everything had always been about them.

After my vertigo resolved, I started biking again with either Alie or Jamie and also took them to run on area tracks. Because they did so well at the Special Olympics, I felt less nervous about letting them run on a track as long as it was fenced in. Shanthy suggested a nearby track and she and her toddler son, David, would sometimes meet us there to run. I'd watch David while Shanthy ran with the boys and Allan stood watch from the opposite side of the track, just to be safe. But the boys did great. Alie would take off ahead of Shanthy and Jamie, but he'd just keep looping the track while Shanthy ran with Jamie at his pace. Jamie loved running with Shanthy. She had such a calming, sweet way with him; she talked to him gently and took his hand in hers. And in races she never rushed him to the starting line. She knew he was content to start and finish in the middle of the pack.

Shanthy soon became more than a coach; she became a friend. She and her husband Rob lived near us in Floral Park. Sometimes she and I met for lunch, and occasionally all four of us went out for dinner while the boys were with their evening therapists. Rob was a runner, as well, so we talked about running and the boys and their sweet David. It was a nice break from focusing on autism, OCD, and on the boys' often challenging behaviors.

———

By the fall of 2006, when the boys were 16 years old, they were running in at least one race a month and usually more often than that. Both Alie and Jamie placed in the National Disability Championship 5K in early October. Alie ran with Kevin and came in first place in

23:43 and Jamie came in third, running with Shanthy in 28:16. They both smiled proudly as medals were placed over their heads. When we arrived home, I hung their medals up with the growing collection on the wall in the den.

Two weeks later, we drove to Oyster Bay for the Oyster Festival 5K. The weather was as glorious as it had been the previous year, the blazing fall colors reminding me once again of my mom. Running had become such a huge part of our lives that it was hard to believe that my mom and dad had never known Alie and Jamie as runners. I also couldn't believe that they had only been running for a year. It seemed as if they'd been doing it forever. Now, we couldn't imagine them *not* running.

That day, Allan and I did what we'd gotten very good at doing: standing on the sideline and screaming the boys' names as they ran by with huge smiles on their faces. After the race Allan and I hugged them, telling them what a great job they did, reinforcing them with high fives. Other runners came over and congratulated them too.

"You got some great athletes here!" one man said, and when we told him that they had severe autism, he shook his head. "Unbelievable."

And it did feel unbelievable. How could these be the same boys who as toddlers had done little more than bang their toys, jump, and flap?

"This is the best thing that's happened to them," Allan said.

"I know," I agreed. I knew it was the happiest Alie and Jamie had ever been. I was filled with gratitude: always for ABA but now also for the leap of faith we took in signing the boys up for Rolling Thunder, for all their coaches, and especially for Kevin and Shanthy and Mike.

14

BY NOVEMBER, ALIE HAD shaved six minutes off his first 5K time and Jamie had shaved off four minutes. They were both getting faster, especially Alie, and especially when he was running with Kevin. But then there were a couple of 5Ks Kevin couldn't run, and in both races the coaches had to link arms with Alie to keep him from taking off without them. Alie practically dragged them the whole way, and at the finish line he looked crestfallen, unable to understand why he wasn't allowed to really run, why he hadn't been able to run the way he ran with Kevin.

After we'd told Kevin about those two races, he called with a proposition: he would train Alie exclusively. We could still meet the Rolling Thunder team at Sunken Meadow so Jamie could run with Shanthy, but Alie would do his own workout with Kevin. And if Kevin couldn't make the Saturday practice time, we'd meet another day and try to coordinate with Shanthy to see if she was available to run with Jamie.

We were thrilled that Kevin wanted to run with Alie more. We knew the consistency would be better for him. Mixing it up had never been easy for Alie, and now he would be able to race the way he was being taught to run in practice.

Kevin shrugged off our gratitude. "Listen," he said. "I'm a runner and I want to run my race. I'm not keen on running someone else's race. Maybe once in a while, but not on a regular basis. With Alie I can do two things at once—run my race and coach Alie at the same time." Then he added, "Alie's a running machine, but there's a lot of room for improvement. I want to see what he can do."

How could we have gotten so lucky?

———

The boys ran in all kinds of weather. A few times during that winter of 2007 when the forecast predicted freezing temperatures and snow, I thought we should skip practice, but Kevin said they needed to learn to run in any weather. We spent some brutally cold mornings at Sunken Meadow or Bethpage State Park, but the boys didn't seem fazed by the temperature, anyway. They started their workout wearing hats and neck warmers and layers, only to strip them off after the first mile or so. I sat in the car with the heat on high.

As always, I laid out their clothes the night before morning runs because they couldn't match a forecast with appropriately warm clothes. And because running was now an obsession for Alie, we had to wait until after they were in bed to get everything ready. If we told Alie that we were running the next morning, he would frenetically run around the house, gathering all our running gear and placing it on the chair in the living room. Then he'd spend an hour methodically spacing and smoothing out the clothes before moving on to arranging his and Jamie's shoes in the den, then filling the cooler. It took forever to get him to calm down and go to sleep. So now we only told them they'd be running when we woke them up in the morning. Alie would still rush through dressing and breakfast, staring at the Nike bag beside him, but at least we had all gotten a good night's sleep.

———

Kevin soon learned that when he ran with Alie, he had to monitor more than just the workout. Before longer runs, he'd have to make sure Alie went to the bathroom. He had to watch Alie closely. Sometimes Alie would become all clogged with mucous because he didn't know how to spit or blow his nose. How could he even breathe? In the summer months, Kevin also had to watch for mosquitos and other insects. If a mosquito or bee landed on Alie's face, he wouldn't swat it away. He was oblivious.

Kevin had to constantly remind Alie to watch where he was going. Alie would often fixate on something—the sun, where we had parked the car, where Kevin left his keys—and he would continue to look in that direction no matter which way the run took them. His head would swivel in that direction the whole run. As long as Alie's head was turned less than ninety degrees, he could use his peripheral vision to find his way, but sometimes he'd be looking back over his shoulder and Kevin would have to say "Where are you going?" and "Straight ahead!" to try to snap Alie out of it.

But Kevin's biggest challenge with Alie was trying to get him to even out his pace so that he could finish a workout as strong as he started it. Because Kevin and Alie were running on their own now, Kevin couldn't send another fast Rolling Thunder runner after Alie if he got away. He would have to run after him himself. Kevin was still faster than Alie so he could always catch him, but it made for an uneven workout.

Kevin started holding on to Alie's shirt and ran like that for the first couple of miles, until Alie was tired out enough to stay with him. But it wasn't long before Kevin developed a hernia from straining like that. Then, for a while, he ran next to Alie with his arm out in front of Alie's chest, switching arms and sides halfway through their workout.

I knew that Alie was capable of learning the rules of running. Like the early days of ABA, it was just a matter of presenting the rules in a way he'd understand it. I thought back to Alie's struggle identifying objects and how it finally worked when we paired the word with a sign. But what was the right way to present this?

One day after practice, I could tell Kevin was frustrated.

"I keep thinking there should be an easy solution," he said.

"Ha!" Allan laughed. "Not with Alie."

"Listen," I said, "If Alie thinks he's not going to be able to run, that would be a huge motivator for him. So maybe every time he sprints out ahead of you, you tell him to stop and walk. And if he doesn't listen, then the workout is done." I hated the thought of Alie not getting his running high and not being able to work off his excess energy, but even more than that I hated the thought of Kevin throwing in the towel. What if he got so frustrated he didn't want to run with Alie anymore? We had to figure out how to make it work.

Kevin learned to be firm with Alie and just say, "Nope, I'm done. I'm sorry. You have to listen." And Alie got a little better. He wouldn't sprint out as far ahead of Kevin. But still, he wasn't responding consistently. By this point, we'd added another day of running to the schedule, meeting Kevin at Bethpage one afternoon a week in addition to Saturday mornings. Allan or I would bike with Jamie while Kevin ran with Alie. The additional day of training seemed to help a little; Alie didn't break away quite as frequently, but it still happened.

The big breakthrough came in the spring of 2007 when Kevin realized that the only way he could really control Alie was to have him run behind him. He'd grab a long branch and run with it sticking out behind him. Alie had to stay behind the branch. Kevin would wiggle it as they ran, trying to maintain Alie's attention *and* enough space between them so Alie wouldn't clip his heels.

After that first practice using the branch, Kevin looked triumphant. "It's not ideal, but at least I can pace us." I couldn't imagine running at all, much less carrying a five-foot branch, but Kevin didn't seem to mind. He was determined to pace Alie.

Both boys were continuing to run in mainstream races, and they were increasing their distances. At the end of March they ran their first 10K, the Nationwide Insurance A.S.P.I.R.E. in Plainview. Jamie ran with Randy and Judy, another Rolling Thunder coach who had been with the team for about three years and, like Shanthy, was sweet and patient. Jamie came in fourth place in his age group at 55:43, and Alie ran with Kevin and came in second in his age group in 43:51, running 7:02 minute miles. And at the beginning of May, in the Great Neck 5K to benefit the Cancer Center for Kids at Winthrop Hospital, Alie placed first overall, running it in 20:30. Kevin was working wonders with Alie despite the challenges inherent in training him.

Jamie still enjoyed a much slower pace than Alie and seemed to run for the love of it. Once he got started, he could run forever. In races, he would still gravitate toward any girl with a swishy ponytail, and he'd stay right behind her, locked into her pace. If she sped up, Jamie would speed up. If she slowed down, Jamie slowed down. He loved water stops, as well, which provided additional social interaction. He would smile and hold out his hand to shake. Then he'd beam when the volunteers smiled back at him and asked how the run was going. He loved that kind of attention. But probably his favorite part of races was the post-race celebration with all the food and music and high fives, all huge reinforcers for Jamie.

Sometimes Jamie got an award for placing in his age group, but if he didn't and Alie did, he'd smile as he watched Alie walk up and get his award. Afterward, when I snapped their picture together, Jamie would reach out to hold Alie's arm. I wasn't sure why he did that. Was he proud of his brother? Proud, too, of himself for running? We couldn't know, but I loved to see that bond between them. It was a glimmer, albeit a tiny one, of what as infants I'd hoped they would be when they grew up: connected, best friends.

Later that month, I received a call from *New York Times* reporter Corey Kilgannon, who had seen an article about the boys and their running in a local Long Island newspaper. He wanted to know how they felt about running, whether they ran together, and how they interacted with one another. I explained that because Alie and Jamie couldn't verbally communicate they couldn't tell us how they felt about running; instead we had to discern it by their expressions and their behavior.

He said he'd love to see the boys run, and Allan and I were both excited. It was one thing for the boys' therapists and coaches and us to think that their running was extraordinary, but it was something else to have the wider world take notice.

Corey met us the following weekend at the Run Day 5K in Hicksville. He was friendly and enthusiastic, talking with Shanthy and Kevin and Allan and me while a photographer took pictures of the boys stretching in the grass. The boys said "hi" when we prompted them to, but they were in their pre-race zone, smiling distantly, anxious for the starting line.

Though the boys were on their best behavior that day, I think Corey was surprised by how severe their autism really was. We had lived with their behaviors for so long that they had become the norm for us. We no longer really thought about it. They were just Alie and Jamie; Jamie and Alie. But what did Corey see? They were certainly no longer the constantly whirling, twirling, flapping boys they had been as young children, but they were clearly not typical. I stared at them warming up, their heads cocked slightly to the side, distant smiles on their faces. Jamie jumped up and down, humming and vocalizing, but Alie just smiled, staring off, excited to run.

They both had a great race. Alie finished with Kevin in 20:53, a 6:44 mile pace, and Jamie finished with Shanthy in 27:45, an 8:45 mile pace. They were beaming as they crossed the finish line, and Corey seemed excited by what they could do.

Allan and I had no idea what to expect from the article, but when the paper arrived on the following Sunday, there they were, front and center in the Long Island Section of the *New York Times*! It felt like a testament to the fact that living with severe autism didn't mean living without talent, without joy. My parents would have loved it.

———

Early that summer, Shanthy left Rolling Thunder because she was pregnant with her second child. We were sad to see her go but knew we'd still be in touch. After that, Jamie ran with one of the other Rolling Thunder coaches. He began running faster 5K times, but he also began developing disruptive behaviors on runs: stopping abruptly or pulling on the coach's arm. Before practices and races, we reminded the coaches to listen for vocalizations or other signs that Jamie was uncomfortable. And if he pulled on their arm, that definitely meant to slow down. That was Jamie's way of communicating.

Because the boys had taken to running the way they did, Randy suggested we raise the bar even higher. "Why don't you see if they can run with the Great Neck South High School cross-country team?"

Participating on a typical high school team wouldn't have crossed our minds before Alie and Jamie began to run, but now they had run 20 races, most of them mainstream, and we knew how much they loved it. What if they could be part of a high school team and run five days a week?

"What do you think?" I asked Allan.

"They'd love it," he said.

"But they'd need one-to-one coaches."

Allan shrugged. "Let's see what the district says. It certainly doesn't hurt to ask."

The boys hadn't participated in any activities through the Great Neck School District, but the district had always been supportive of their needs. I had heard so many horror stories from other parents with children with autism and other special needs about how they had had to fight for placement for their children or fight for other supports like home therapy hours. Over the years I had attended regular CSE (Committee on Special Education) meetings, of course, in which Mary or Randy and the boys' teacher from Genesis and I would meet with the head of the Special Education Department and a district psychologist or social worker, and we'd review the boys' progress and needs. But there was never a question about the fact that they were exactly where they needed to be at Genesis. And the district approved any request I made: home therapy, parent training hours, new AAC devices for Alie as he progressed from simpler to more elaborate devices through the years. Even the district transportation staff that took Alie and Jamie to and from Genesis every school day was amazing.

But we needed a proposal to present to the district, so Randy suggested we meet with Linda Meyer, the co-founder of the Alpine Learning Center, a renowned ABA-based school in New Jersey. I knew Linda and loved her enthusiasm, and her area of specialty was studying how exercise affected those with autism. "She's the perfect person to help you," Randy said.

And she was right. We met with Linda at Eden II on Staten Island, and she was so excited about the possibility of the boys running with Great Neck South. She helped us craft the proposal to the district in which we outlined the boys' needs and made the case for hiring two one-to-one coaches for Alie and Jamie for the season.

We hoped that Kevin would be interested in being Alie's coach, and when we asked him he was thrilled. "Yes! And to have the boys running every day will be amazing!" Kevin followed the local high school sports teams, so he was already familiar with South's team, and he was also a Certified USA Track and Field coach. He would be ideal for the position, and since his work was flexible, he could make the daily practices, which were from 3:00 to 5:00 PM every weekday.

The meeting with the district was seamless, and Damon, the South High cross-country coach, welcomed Alie and Jamie to the team. Kevin was hired as Alie's one-to-one coach, and Hudson, a teacher in the district, was hired as Jamie's one-to-one coach. Hudson didn't have a background in autism, but he was a great runner, was warm and friendly, and he listened closely when we explained Jamie's lack of ability to communicate and described signs that he might want to slow down.

The season started at the end of August, which was perfect because the boys were off from school for a week, so we could transition them into the new running schedule before we had to transition them into the new school year.

The night before their first practice after we had gotten them in bed, I sat on the couch with Allan.

"I can't believe how this worked out," I said. "Especially that Kevin will be Alie's one-to-one."

Allan shook his head, smiling. "I never would have guessed it."

Even though we both knew something would always come up with the boys, as it always did, for a moment it was nice to celebrate how far we'd come. Yes, the boys still had severe autism; yes, they were still nonverbal; yes, they still had sometimes debilitating OCD; but they were doing something they loved, and they were going to be doing it with their peers at their home high school.

Allan leaned down and kissed me, and I smiled and kissed him back.

———

I took Alie and Jamie to practice each afternoon so Allan could rest in a quiet house, something he still needed to do daily in order to manage his MS symptoms. And when they started back at Genesis, they changed into their running clothes at school and the district bus picked them up at 2:15 PM and dropped them at the high school, where Kevin and I would meet them, take them to the bathroom, and then go to the field to warm up with the team.

I loved those afternoons at the high school. I sat at the bottom of a steep hill where the team warmed up and watched as they stretched and did jumping jacks, push ups, and sit ups. The boys had learned some of these exercises when they were in the PALS basketball program, so for the most part they were able to keep up as long Kevin and Hudson prompted them. Then they would take off as a team across the wide fields toward the wooded trail.

Kevin was worried about the boys jumping from running two days to five days a week, so the first week they only ran four out of the five practices. Kevin and Hudson moderated the workouts, as well; if the team was doing 10 half-mile repeats on the track, they'd have the boys do two or three of them and then come sit one out next to me before jumping back in.

————

After practice, I'd take them home, get them changed, and set out a snack for them. Then they'd spend the next couple of hours with their therapists, who tried to get them out into the community as much as possible. Both of them seemed to love their new schedule.

Allan and I occasionally had dinner together while the boys were with their therapists, but often we did chores around the house or ran errands. Theresa had left to open her own business, an organic market and restaurant. We were happy that she was following her dream, but we missed her.

I often had work from the day that I needed to wrap up, as well, or emails to send to the home or school teams about the boys. Alie still had numerous behavioral issues that we had to troubleshoot. His pica was an ongoing problem and he'd begun flapping his hands and snapping his wrists again. But though these behaviors were a problem at home and school, they vanished when Alie ran. He was calm and focused, and Kevin said he seemed like he was in heaven at practice, surrounded by so many other fast runners.

Jamie seemed to enjoy running with the team, as well, but sometimes he'd pull on Hudson during runs. He was trying to tell Hudson to slow down or stop or that he was uncomfortable, and if Hudson didn't pick up on that, Jamie would get even more upset. One time he went down on his knees and pulled Hudson to the ground with him. Hudson was used to coaching a team and pushing the kids to run faster. He quickly learned Jamie's way: no pushing.

————

It was the beginning of September now, and the weather was perfect. One afternoon, the team had done a longer run across campus and through the woods, and I was standing at the bottom of the hill chatting with Damon, waiting for them to return. Finally we saw the first runners come over the hill, and they were flying, Alie right behind them with Kevin.

Alie looked like he was sprinting full out, but suddenly I realized that there was something off with his gait.

I turned to Damon. "Is Alie limping?"

Damon watched the runners for a moment. "It looks like he is. Something's not right."

My stomach dropped. *No, no, no.*

A minute later, when Alie came to a stop in front of me, he was smiling his usual huge smile.

"Are you okay, Alie? Does anything hurt?" I asked, though I'm not sure why. I knew he wouldn't be able to tell me.

Alie just kept smiling.

Then Kevin was there and said he thought Alie was favoring one leg on that final hill.

"Alie, come here. Sit down. I want to see your foot." I patted the ground next to me and Alie sat down. I unlaced his running shoes, hoping it was nothing. It had to be nothing. The season just started. But when I pulled off his right sock, the top of his foot was red.

"Oh, no," said Kevin. He looked sick to his stomach. "I was trying to be so careful, easing him in."

But of course it wasn't Kevin's fault. The trails around the high school were full of roots and rocks. He could have stepped down on something wrong, especially with his heavy footfalls.

One of the boys' therapists, Debbie, came over to help. Sometimes on the days she was scheduled to work with the boys in the afternoon, she came to watch them practice with me. Debbie was a runner, too, and she was so excited that the boys were able to run five days a week now.

Debbie and I helped Alie and Jamie to the car, and as soon as we got home I called the doctor. Alie's arch had started to swell, so Debbie held an ice pack to it. He ordinarily wouldn't have remained still, even after a strenuous run, but he sat quietly next to her on the couch. I think he knew something was wrong, but he kept smiling, as if he was saying, "Please help me so I can get back to running."

On the phone, the doctor said he thought it sounded like a stress fracture. Allan had heard us come in and met me in the kitchen. I covered the phone with my hand and mouthed "stress fracture."

"What? Oh no!" he whispered. That was exactly how I felt. Things had been going so well for Alie on the cross-country team, and now this.

I took Alie in that evening for an X-ray, but it was too soon to see anything definitive, so the doctor ordered an MRI. But how would I keep Alie calm and still enough for an MRI? We had to at least try it, though, or we wouldn't know how to treat his foot.

I called for an appointment and also asked to speak with the technician to explain Alie's autism and inability to sit still. He said they'd give it a try, so the next day, I took Alie in for an MRI. I brought his iPod with his favorite music, but even with that and me sitting right next to him, he became agitated and began moving around.

They were only able to complete about half of it, but it was enough. Alie had "prominent intramedullary bone marrow edema extending throughout the second metatarsal bone compatible with an acute stress fracture." Eight weeks of recovery. He'd be out of cross-country the whole season.

All of us were devastated. Kevin felt horrible, though neither he nor Damon thought Alie had been running long enough at the increased mileage to cause a stress fracture. He must have come down hard on his foot and jarred it.

Kevin was committed to the team, and all the runners loved him, so after Alie was hurt, he continued on as an assistant coach and took over as Jamie's one-to-one coach. Hudson stayed on to coach the other runners, and I think he was probably relieved not to have to try to decipher Jamie's distress signals.

Kevin had never really run with Jamie, and after that first practice he smiled, shaking his head. "Well, Alie and Jamie may be identical twins, but they couldn't be more different." Kevin had to modify his training and slow everything way down. But Kevin quickly became familiar with Jamie's behaviors and his way of communicating.

"When Jamie wants to slow down," Kevin said after practice one day, "he says, 'Okay, okay.' At first I didn't know what that meant, so I didn't slow down. So then Jamie put his hand on my arm and pulled. I realized that was my second warning. If I didn't respond to that, I realized he'd get upset and go down."

I felt badly that Kevin was having to run so much slower than he would have liked, so much slower than he had been running with Alie, but I was relieved that Jamie was running with someone so in tune with him.

In the meets, instead of lining up with all the other runners on the starting line and getting out fast, Jamie insisted on standing 20 yards back. He was sensitive to loud noises, and the blaring horn startled him at the beginning of each race. But Kevin and Jamie would eventually work their way up into the race. Jamie was running his best 5K times that season. If there were a hundred boys competing, Jamie would beat at least 15 of them. But it didn't matter to Jamie. He wasn't interested in competing. He ran at his own pace and was excited to see us at the finish line.

Alie took the bus home from school without Jamie, while Jamie was picked up earlier and dropped at the high school for practice, which threw Alie off a little. Why had this schedule he loved changed? Why couldn't he run? But although Alie wasn't able to burn off any of his excess energy, which increased his anxiety, he was, for the most part, subdued. I think he was sad.

At home, Allan and I both babied him, hugging him and giving him a ton of attention, not only to cheer him up but also to make sure he stayed off his foot as much as possible. He was compliant, slowing down when we told him to slow down, never fussing in the shower when we had to wrap his soft cast in plastic so it wouldn't get wet. And if he started to hobble through the house too quickly, we just had to remind him about his foot and tell him that if he wanted to run he had to heal. He'd slow down immediately. I felt so bad for him.

———

We usually left Alie at home with one of his therapists when Jamie had a meet because we thought it would confuse and upset him to be there and not be able to run, but we did take him to Jamie's last meet of the season. Alie stood next to me motionless, watching all the runners line up at the start, then take off at the sound of the gun. Allan and I were cheering and clapping for Jamie, so Alie imitated us and clapped, as well. He was smiling, too, and I think he enjoyed being a part of that environment again. But when I looked over at him as the runners flew by us, his eyes were full of tears.

My heart sank. I didn't remember him ever crying before. Not ever.

"Oh Alie," I said, as I put my arm around him. "Don't worry. You'll be running again soon, as soon as your foot's all better."

He looked at me and reached down and touched his foot. He had been wearing a soft cast for weeks already, so I think he understood, but still, it broke my heart to see him so sad.

15

JAMIE FINISHED OUT HIS cross-country season strong, and both he and Alie earned Varsity letters, even though Alie had been out practically the whole season. I was grateful to Damon for including him. We were invited to the end of the season celebration in the high school gymnasium. I couldn't be there because of a work meeting I couldn't reschedule, but Allan videotaped the ceremony as he sat among the other parents in the bleachers. Jamie and Alie stood next to two of our home therapists, who held their hands as they waited for their names to be called. When Damon handed each of the boys their certificate and their orange and blue letter "S," their teammates and all their parents burst into applause. When I watched it on our video player later, I had to blink away my tears.

———

After the cross-country season ended, Jamie resumed running with Rolling Thunder on Saturday mornings at Sunken Meadow. But we heard more and more reports from his coaches that he seemed agitated on the runs, pulling on them or vocalizing loudly, clearly distressed even after they eased up on the pace.

When those behaviors started, Jamie was already upset and it was often difficult to calm him down, so the key was to redirect him or slow down *before* he became anxious. That was tricky, however, because the signs were subtle and weren't consistent. Sometimes he'd vocalize loudly, sometimes softly. Sometimes he'd develop a stuttering step, as if his foot was catching in midair. The signs changed, though, so they were easy to misinterpret. And if a coach redirected Jamie when he really didn't need to be redirected, he'd react as well, feeling, we guessed, admonished. It was a delicate balance, and Allan and I knew it was a lot to expect of the coaches.

We were also trying to balance speed versus joy. We wanted to keep Jamie with a fast coach because we knew he was capable of running at that pace, but we also wanted him to enjoy the run and not feel pressured. Ray was the Rolling Thunder coach who got the fastest times from Jamie, but in doing so he also pushed Jamie more than some of the other coaches. At the end of August, Ray had gotten Jamie to run a 25:00 5K, a PR (personal record) at an 8:03 pace. Then at the beginning of October, Jamie came in second place in his age group in the National Disability Championship 5K, running it in 26:23. But after that race, Ray said he'd had some vocalizations. Jamie seemed fine at the finish line, though perhaps a little less euphoric than usual.

On the way home, Allan and I were both quiet. It had been a good race for Jamie, but we knew we needed to better help the coaches identify warning signs. But maybe that was too much to ask. I reached back and patted Jamie's knee. He was humming along to his iPod but smiled when I touched him.

Alie was staring out the window, tracking the flittering light through the trees. He had looked so sad again when the gun went off at the start of the race. That morning Allan and I had talked about one of us staying back with him, but it was a big race for Rolling Thunder and we wanted Alie to be part of it, even if only as a spectator. We had explained to Alie that he wouldn't be able to run and he seemed to understand. He hadn't gotten upset when Jamie put on his running clothes and he didn't.

But he became agitated and began pulling on my arm when we got to the race, and I tried to leave him with Allan and Jamie while I went up to the registration table to get Jamie's bib. Alie always went up with me to get the bibs—he loved every aspect of race day—so finally I agreed to let him come with me.

Lenny, one of the Rolling Thunder coaches, was handling registrations and he smiled when he saw us. "Alie, you'll be running again in no time!"

But the whole thing was too much for Alie. He grabbed a bib from the table and frantically pressed it to his chest.

"Oh, Alie, I'm sorry. You can't run today," I said.

"That's heartbreaking," said Lenny. "He wants to run so badly."

It *was* heartbreaking, and I realized it had been a mistake to bring him. He just didn't understand why he couldn't do the thing he loved.

I finally was able to get him to put down the bib, but as we walked away he was clearly distressed. "Soon," I'd reassured him. "You'll get to run again very soon."

We were almost home when Allan said, "I'm going to start running with Jamie."

"What?" I said, turning to him.

Allan glanced at me, his eyebrows raised. "*I'm* going to run with Jamie."

I'd heard him the first time, of course; I just didn't believe it. "You can't run with Jamie!" I said, exasperated. "You haven't run in years! You'll slow him down. And what about your MS?"

"Actually, I've been doing a lot of reading, and more and more the research is saying that exercise helps with MS symptoms."

I was doubtful. Though Allan biked alongside the boys and we went for long walks with them, I couldn't imagine him running a 5K or something longer—especially fast enough to keep up with Jamie.

Not to mention that intense exertion seemed to exacerbate his MS symptoms, not help them. "I don't think so, Allan."

"Listen," Allan said, waving his hand in the air. "Jamie's been running with all these different coaches. He starts out fine, then has these behaviors. It's a lot to expect them to really understand Jamie. I think I can do better as his coach."

I sighed. He definitely needed someone who had insight into his behaviors and knew how to read him. "Maybe we just need to go over the warning signs again," I said. "I think they can manage him if we just keep working on it."

I glanced back at Jamie, who was oblivious that he was the subject of our conversation.

Allan shook his head. "Why are you so resistant to me running with him?"

Why was I so resistant? Was it because then I'd be alone at the finish line and need to corral Alie by myself after the race? Or that I knew Allan wouldn't be fast enough and Jamie would be held back? Or was I jealous that he would be running with Jamie and I wouldn't be? I wasn't sure.

"We've always said safety is first. You're always saying that." He pulled into our driveway and turned off the car. "But it's not safe for Jamie to run with someone who doesn't understand him. *I* can handle his anxiety. *I* know the signs. And it doesn't matter if he runs slower with me."

"Of course safety is always first," I responded, irritated. "But I'm worried about you too. It might be too much."

"I'll work up to it," Allan said. "I'll start running on my own and when I feel ready, I can run with the team, then Jamie." He slid his sunglasses onto his head. "Sure, Jamie might run slower with me. But he'll be in his comfort zone. He's not like Alie. He doesn't care about competing, anyway."

I couldn't argue with that. Allan was right. And I knew I wouldn't be able to dissuade him once his mind was made up.

"Okay," I finally said, shaking my head as I opened my car door. "Let's see how it goes."

Allan began to run a couple of times a week during the day while I was working and the boys were at school. "It's hard," he admitted. "But I'll get there." He started out running through the hilly streets of Great Neck. He went out in the morning and tracked his course, each day adding additional blocks to it. He was very pleased with himself and would tell me how far he ran each day: a mile, a mile and a half, two miles.

Though he was only increasing his runs by a few blocks each time, he was excited about it. He still had regular leg cramps and his body ached at night, but he was clearly proud that he was working toward his goal of running with Jamie. He became obsessed with getting his runs in.

I started to think more and more about what was right for Jamie, and I began to realize that this really *was* the best idea, to have Allan run with him. The priority was to keep it fun and safe for Jamie; his speed was secondary. So I began to encourage Allan, making sure he was able to carve out the time to run.

———

At the beginning of November, after eight long weeks of no running, Alie was finally cleared to run again. We were relieved but also concerned that he'd reinjure himself. He had become easier to pace because he'd learned that if he wanted to run with Kevin, he had to stay behind him, but Kevin was worried that because he hadn't run in so long, he'd try to sprint all out as soon as they were on the trail.

Before that first practice back, I had laid Alie's running clothes out with Jamie's in the den, and when Alie came downstairs, I showed him his schedule, which listed "running" just after "breakfast." He smiled as he put on his clothes and shoes, but he seemed hesitant, as if he didn't trust that it was really going to happen. He didn't try to rush Jamie through breakfast or out the door. He just stood at the door to the garage, watching as Jamie slowly put on his hat.

We drove out to Sunken Meadow to meet the team, and everyone was excited to see Alie again, giving him high fives and welcoming him back. He smiled and I could tell how happy he was. Jamie stretched with a group of runners, and we reminded the coach to take it slow with him and to ease up further if he started vocalizing or had any stutter steps.

We watched the team head out across the field while Kevin and Alie took off in the opposite direction.

"I hope he's okay," Allan said, watching Kevin and Alie disappear onto the trail.

"Me too." I hated the thought of having to keep Alie from running any longer than we'd already had to.

But when Kevin and Alie appeared 25 minutes later, he seemed great, his gait steady.

"Alie would have liked to keep going," Kevin said. "But we'll take it slow. But he did great. He stayed right with me."

Jamie had a great run that day, as well. He looped slowly through the woods and across the meadow and was smiling when we helped him into his sweatshirt after practice. "No behaviors at all," one of the coaches reported, giving Jamie a high five. "He loved it."

———

Kevin ran with Alie twice a week leading up to Thanksgiving and suggested that the four-mile Townwide Fund of Huntington Thanksgiving Day Race would be a perfect comeback race for Alie. Jamie really seemed to like trail races, and we had already registered him to run a 5K trail run with Rolling Thunder the Sunday after Thanksgiving, so

Allan and I agreed that I'd take Alie to the Townwide race while he stayed home with Jamie to cook the turkey.

When we arrived in Huntington, Alie was beaming. Typically at the start of the race, he rushed to get his bib and pulled on me until I pinned it on for him, then he'd want to move right to the starting line. But that day he seemed calm, and I wished I knew what he was thinking, how he really felt.

"Are you excited to run?"

"Yesss!" he said.

But he calmly held my hand as we waited for Kevin to arrive, and then they went off for a short warm-up jog.

As I waited for them, a couple we'd bumped into at a number of races waved to me.

"Hey, we haven't seen you out in a while. How are the boys?"

"Great," I said, smiling. "But Alie's been out with a stress fracture for the last two months. This is his first race since August."

"Ohh. Ouch. We hope it goes well!"

"Thank you!" I said, touched by their concern. But we had already realized that that's how the Long Island running community was: warm and welcoming. And the more people we met at races, the more people there were cheering for Alie and Jamie at the finish line.

When Kevin and Alie returned, I walked with them to the starting line and gave Alie a quick kiss and told him to have a great run. He looked more focused and happier than I'd seen him since his injury. Then the gun sounded and they were off.

The wind was chilly off Huntington Harbor, but I didn't mind. The sun was bright and Alie was racing again. Since my mom died, November had been a hard month for me, especially since my parents used to come to our house to celebrate Thanksgiving with us before they left to spend the winter in Florida. But though I still missed them terribly, I knew we had a lot for which to be thankful. I stood in the throng of spectators, rubbed my gloved hands together, and thought about Allan's signature turkey dinner. We would gather around our dining room table together and Allan and I would raise our glasses in gratitude.

I watched the runners coming down the hill to the finish line, hoping that Alie was having a good race. And then I saw him approach in his Thanksgiving Day race shirt, Kevin right behind him. All Kevin had to do as they neared the finish line was just move to the side a little, and say, "Go, Alie!" and Alie would sprint his way across the line. Today was no different. He was intent on the finish line, and I could tell he was in his Zen place. I got chills watching him run by me as I screamed his name.

Alie finished in 28:29, 84th out of 1,002 runners. Kevin didn't want to push him too hard, so his 7:08 pace was slower than usual, but I knew he was back.

———

Allan was also feeling more confident in his running. By the end of November he was running a couple of miles a few times a week, and he asked me to register him when I registered the boys for the annual HoHoHo 5K run in mid-December.

In early December he also started running with Rolling Thunder on Saturdays. He was running a 12-minute pace or slower, so he didn't run with Jamie during practice, but instead with some of the slower athletes on the team. He'd finish the workout elated, though the trails were difficult for him to navigate. Allan had slight drop foot due to his MS, and it was hard for him to lift the front of his feet high enough to clear roots and rocks on the path. The more fatigued he became, the harder it was for his brain to send the right signals to his feet, and he'd frequently trip and fall down. I know it was frustrating for him, but not frustrating enough to give up running, especially because Jamie seemed to love having Allan there even though they weren't running together.

As Jamie took off, Allan would yell, "I'll be running too Jamie, right behind you!" Jamie would start off but look back at Allan, trailing along at the end of the pack. And when Jamie's workout was finished, he would stare at the trail until Allan appeared out of the woods with the other runners.

Allan had always been determined; whenever he set his mind to something, he always accomplished it. So I started to feel excited, too, imagining him running races with Jamie. It would be great for both of them.

Practicing with the team appealed to Allan's social nature, and he ended up loving it. Most of the teenagers with whom he ran were high functioning, so they would talk the whole way—sports, school—and Allan would regale them with stories of his own teenage years.

I knew how much he would have loved to have that kind of relationship with Alie and Jamie, and I finally understood that Allan's desire to run with Jamie went way beyond safety. Safety might have been the impetus to get him running, but running would also provide a way for Allan and Jamie to connect; to share something with each other.

Over the years I'd often thought about what autism had stolen from the boys: they would never go on a date or make love or get married. They would never go to college or choose professions about which they were passionate. They would never become parents themselves. I had mourned those losses for them. And I had mourned the fact that we would never experience those things with them either.

But Alie and Jamie were much more affectionate than many kids with severe autism, and I knew they loved us and felt safe with us, so I never felt I had to mourn that special mother-child connection. We *were* connected. But I realized how much we still missed out on and, later, what Allan specifically missed out on: he would never be able to teach Alie or Jamie to drive; he would never be able to talk to them about girlfriends, college, politics, or his own childhood. That kind of a relationship would never be possible. What he *could* do was share something else with Jamie; he could run with him. So despite the setbacks he faced on the trails because of his MS, Allan kept at it.

At the HoHoHo in mid-December, he lined up behind Alie and Jamie and their coaches for his first 5K ever. Like the two previous HoHoHo races, it was cold day, but this year the race was held at a new location: the Old Bethpage Village Restoration, a 19th-century village re-created on 209 acres of land. They would run on dirt paths and roads through the village and surrounding area, but the roads were full of ruts and patches of ice, and I was nervous that one of them would slip and fall.

Thankfully, they were all fine. First Alie and Kevin came in, then Jamie and Judy. Then we all waited for Allan, who smiled and waved to us as he came around the bend, clearly elated. He lifted his fist and pumped the air as he ran past, finishing in 37:40, a 12:08 minute pace. I laughed, knowing that he'd be running with Jamie in no time.

16

AT THE BEGINNING OF 2008, when the boys were 17, Alie developed new OCD behaviors around music and his iPod. Music had always been something that soothed him, but now he'd pick up his iPod, fast-forward through every song, then put it down on the ottoman and stare at it while he karate chopped the couch, then stomped his feet on the hardwood floor. We were especially worried about his feet—that he'd hurt himself again and not be able to run. We were also worried that the behavior would carry over to school. I met with Mary and she developed a behavior plan so that the school and home staff and Allan and I would all be on the same page in dealing with it. As always, we'd try to interrupt the patterns as soon as possible in order to break the chain of behaviors. Then we'd redirect Alie, replacing the problematic behavior with a more appropriate one. But if we didn't redirect him in time and he began the ritual, we couldn't stop him; if we tried to interrupt him he'd grab or hit or bite. It was exhausting, trying to stay ahead of this new obsession, but I also knew that just as in all high-intensity times Alie must be suffering. He probably didn't really want to do these things; he was compelled to do them.

But even with all of these new behaviors, the new year somehow filled me with optimism. Allan and the boys were running, and Allan had begun to run occasionally with Jamie. They were slow, but Jamie seemed happy. The future felt bright. I was looking forward to a year of cheering on my family at the finish line.

But then, in late January, my breast ultrasound showed a small lump. I wasn't too worried about it because I assumed it was a fibroadenoma, the same kind of benign mass I'd had a few years earlier. I went in for a core needle biopsy, just as I had before, and afterward I ran some errands and then went home to try to get a little work done. I was still working for Eden II and I had to catch up on a few emails.

A couple of days later on a Friday I was sitting across from my naturopath, Dr. Stills, in her office when my cell phone rang. I had been seeing Dr. Stills regularly since my debilitating bout of vertigo. I still experienced some spinning when I bent down or turned too quickly, but the diet and supplements had seemed to help, and overall I had more energy.

I pulled my phone from my purse and saw that it was Nassau Radiologic Group.

"I'm sorry," I said to Dr. Stills, holding up my phone.

She nodded. "Go ahead."

"Hello?" I said.

It was the radiologist. She said hello, then paused for a moment. "I'm sorry to have to tell you this, Robyn." Another pause. "But the biopsy shows a malignancy."

A malignancy. Did she just say malignancy?

"What?" I said.

"The biopsy," she repeated. "It's malignant."

My chest tightened. Malignant. Malignant.

An MRI was scheduled for Monday, but I don't know what else she or I said. I hung up and just sat there, cradling my phone in my hands, suddenly freezing. Then I began to shake.

"What?" said Dr. Stills, standing and moving toward me.

"It's malignant," I managed.

"Oh Robyn, I'm so sorry." She reached for me and pulled me into a hug, gently rubbing my back. "I'm here. I will help you through this."

For a moment I felt safe there in her arms, but then I felt my throat constrict. *What will this mean for us? What if I die? Who will take care of the boys?* Questions that I couldn't answer and couldn't bear to contemplate detonated like tiny bombs in my head.

Still holding back the tears, I said, "Thank you. I'll call you when I know more." And then I ran from her office into the parking lot. The brittle winter air made me feel even colder. *Malignant. Cancer. This can't be.* It was only when I was sitting in my car that I began to cry, long wracking sobs.

My biggest fear—the thing I thought about every night before I fell asleep and first thing in the morning—was that Allan and I would die before we could get the boys settled somewhere safe, somewhere they could be happy. What would happen to them when we weren't here to take care of them, to talk sweetly to them, to do all the loving things that parents do?

Now that fear landed like a brick in my chest. I could not leave my sons. Allan wouldn't be able to do it on his own.

———

Somehow I got myself home. I called Allan on my way and stumbled through the news, and he was waiting by the door, his arms open, fear etched into the lines on his face, which was white, as if all the blood had drained from him. I fell into his arms and we both cried, clinging to each other, not believing it, yet knowing that it was really happening.

I felt weak. "I have to sit," I said, and Allan led me to the couch. Cold winter afternoon light poured in the windows. I didn't even know where to begin. All I knew was that I had a malignant tumor and I'd need surgery, just as my mom had. I started to cry again, and Allan hugged me tightly.

"We'll figure this out," he said, and even though we were both terrified and I couldn't silence the questions in my mind, I knew we would—we had to. Since the boys were diagnosed with autism, I had been the one in control. I was the one who handled the boys' home therapy, the school meetings, all correspondence with their school and doctors—everything. I looked at my phone. We had less than an hour before they would get home from school. I needed to pull myself together and make a plan.

I looked at Allan and said, "Kostroff. Dr. Karen Kostroff. She's the one I want to see." I had heard her name before and remembered seeing her name in a *New York Magazine*'s Best Doctors issue. She was the Chief of Breast Surgery for the North Shore–Long Island Jewish Health System, and I'd only heard glowing reviews—especially that she had a gentle bedside manner.

I went to the computer and pulled up her office number, and I called and explained that the biopsy showed cancer and that I had an MRI scheduled for Monday. The receptionist was kind but direct. "I'm very sorry to hear that," she said. "It's great that you already have an MRI scheduled, because Dr. Kostroff will want to see that." She paused. "She's in surgery on Tuesdays, but we can get you in at 10:00 AM on Wednesday."

"Oh, thank you," I said, feeling a small loosening in my chest, grateful I'd get to see her so soon.

Allan went into the kitchen and boiled some water for green tea and set out plates and snacks for the boys. It was Friday so they had therapy, but until the therapists came, we tag-teamed it. I had to begin and keep Alie on a schedule of activities *before* he started with his iPod, which meant I couldn't leave his side from the time he got home until his therapists arrived. Allan kept Jamie busy in the other room, because he was still easily upset by Alie's obsessive behaviors.

I had a sudden need to hear Ruth's voice, so I dialed her number.

"Hi, Rob!" she said. I felt bad for dropping this bomb on her, but I needed her to know. After Allan, and since my parents died, she was one of the first people I turned to during a crisis. I told her about the diagnosis.

"Oh honey! I'm so sorry." I could hear the concern in her voice, but I couldn't afford to let myself cry anymore. Not now. Not with the boys almost home.

"I have an MRI Monday and an appointment with a surgeon on Wednesday," I said.

"Good," she said. "Good. I'm here, whatever you need."

I knew she would be, as always.

"But you know, Robyn, you're going to have to put yourself first in order to make it through this."

"Hmm," I said. *Put myself first*. It reminded me of the pre-flight safety talk they always gave on airplanes, how you needed to put on your own mask first and then your child's. I got that, and I knew I should do it in my daily life—take time for myself, sometimes put myself first—but that wasn't my reality. It wasn't how I worked. Since the boys were little, they always came first, and then after their diagnosis, nothing else mattered. There was a part of me that had always blamed myself for their autism, thought that it must have been something I had done. I knew that was crazy, but I couldn't shake it completely, and it helped to stay focused on them, to always put them first. I couldn't imagine doing it any other way.

"I'm serious," Ruth said. "I have some meditation tapes that I know will help. I'll bring them over this weekend."

"Okay," I said. "Love you."

I knew she was right; I'd have to figure out a way to take care of myself in order to make it through this, but I didn't know what that would look like. Before I became a mother, I could do that—put myself first. Allan and I traveled, I took horseback riding lessons, and I loved to play the piano and read. There was an ease with which I moved through the world. But for almost two decades, everything about my life had been about caring and advocating for Alie and Jamie. How could I possibly change that now?

When Alie and Jamie got home from school, it was easy not to think about the cancer. I was right there next to Alie for the next couple of hours, redirecting him, trying as always to stay one step ahead of his OCD.

That night, after Allan and I put the boys to bed, I laid out their clothes for their morning run, then shed my own clothes and stepped into the shower. And it was as if the hot water released something in me. I began to cry quietly, enveloped in steam, fear bubbling again to the surface. How could my body now be host to something dangerous, something deadly? I had been taking such good care of myself. I had been eating right. I stared down at my breasts, streaming with water, unable to imagine myself without them. What if I needed a mastectomy? How would I reside in a body that was no longer my own? I gave myself a mental shake. If I had to do it, I would. Of course. The boys. What would happen to them if I wasn't here?

I thought of my mom and her cancer. When she had been diagnosed just after my dad died, I remember how stoic she'd been. She seemed so calm, saying, "Whatever will be will be." But I couldn't possibly feel that way. My mom had been almost 80 years old and a widow. I was only 51, and I had too much at stake. My family needed me. I wished Mom were still alive. I needed her. She'd know what to say to cut through my worrying.

I let the hot water beat on my shoulders, loosening the knots that always resided there. As I dried off I decided that I would be strong. I'd do anything it took to beat this. Some women beat it; lots of them did. I decided I was going to be one of them.

——

The next morning after the boys were dressed and had breakfast, we headed to Bethpage State Park to meet Kevin. Allan had started to run some practices with Jamie, and though Jamie was running much slower than he had before, he wasn't having any meltdowns.

Kevin was stretching against his car in the parking lot when we arrived and he gave us a wave as we pulled up next to him. When we got out of the car, Kevin gave Alie and Jamie high fives.

"How are you?" Kevin asked.

"We've had some bad news," Allan said, nodding at me.

"Oh?" Kevin furrowed his brow.

And then it was out—the biopsy, the MRI, and follow-up with Dr. Kostroff in a few days. The boys fidgeted next to me as I spoke, and I knew they were anxious to run. Kevin looked worried. I hated to tell him about the cancer. His sister had died of breast cancer, which is what brought him and Leslie back to Long Island.

"Oh Robyn, I'm so sorry." He hugged me and then Allan.

Alie began kicking the ground next to me, and I knew he was getting impatient.

"Thank you," I said to Kevin. "And sorry to drop this on you. Go run."

I stood in the parking lot and watched Alie run off in one direction with Kevin, Allan and Jamie in the other. I knew the boys could sense my stress, and I was relieved that they were now off doing what they loved. My bike was leaning against the back of the car because I had planned to ride while they were running, but now I didn't feel up for biking. Instead I pulled out my phone and headed for the open field, my shoes breaking through the thin layer of icy snow.

As soon as Edie heard my voice, she knew something was wrong. When Mom was in the hospital and I would call with daily reports, I had the same shakiness in my voice.

"I have breast cancer," I said.

"Oh no, Rob. What happened?" Her voice dropped.

It all spilled out, and although I tried to compose myself, I couldn't steady my voice.

"What's next?"

I told her about the MRI and the appointment with Dr. Kostroff.

"What can I do to help? I can come stay."

I so appreciated the offer, the thought of my sister dropping her life to come be with me, but I knew it didn't make sense. Our biggest challenge would be the boys. If I had to spend time in the hospital—I had no idea what lay ahead—Allan would need help with Alie and Jamie. And the only people who could really manage them were their therapists and teachers.

"Well, let me know what I can do," Edie said. I could hear the heaviness in her voice.

"I will," I said. "I love you."

"Love you, too."

Over the next hour, I called friend after friend, and each one offered to help with anything I needed. I called Randy and she offered to take the boys overnight, and Joanne said not to worry about taking time off work. I called my childhood friend, Brenda, and she offered to come stay with us. And I knew that our home therapists would all pitch in and work extra hours if we needed the help. I was buoyed by all of their love and support, but still I felt myself floundering. How would we make it through this while we juggled the boys and their needs?

"We'll make it through," Allan said later that day. "We're going to beat this." He sounded strong, but I knew he was as frightened as I was.

Just as my dad had done when Allan was diagnosed with MS and when the boys were diagnosed with autism, Allan quickly shifted into research mode. He paged through our stacks of natural healing books, and on Sunday morning he went to the supermarket and came back with bags of groceries—immune system boosters and antioxidants— and made me the first of what would become hundreds of smoothies chocked full of ginger, kiwi, turmeric, black currant jelly—anything to improve my cell health. Even though we didn't yet know what we were up against, he was on a mission to make sure I did everything I could do to increase my chances of survival.

On Sunday afternoon, Ruth stopped by with a bag full of things for me. She hugged me close and then we went to sit down on the sofa. The boys' therapists had taken them for a walk into downtown Great Neck, and Allan went into the kitchen to make us some tea and give us some space.

Ruth set the bag on the coffee table and looked at me. "We've known each other since the boys were little," she said quietly. "And I know you're fierce—you'd do anything for your family." She reached inside her bag and pulled out several books. "But now it's time to think about yourself."

She handed me *Peace Is Every Step* by Thich Nhat Hanh. Ruth was a believer in meditation and spirituality, and she practiced regularly. I certainly wasn't opposed to meditation—I had always considered myself a spiritual person—but I never seemed to have time to try it.

She pulled out a few mediation CDs from the bag, as well, and said, "These will help."

I could feel the familiar excuse—I don't have time—on the tip of my tongue, and I'm sure Ruth could tell it was coming. She pursed her lips. "Rob, this is a really stressful time. I know things are hard with Alie right now, and now to be dealing with this. But if you don't take care of yourself, things are going to get worse for the boys. You know how in tune they are with emotions. They know when you're upset. And when you're upset, they're upset. It always leads to behavioral problems."

"I know," I said, nodding. They could feel my anxiety all weekend, both seeming more agitated than usual. And the last thing I needed was more challenging behaviors right now. "Thank you," I said, smiling at my friend. "I'll try them. I will."

She made me promise and offered to come and stay with the boys whenever we needed.

———

That night after the boys were asleep, I got into bed and opened *Peace Is Every Step*. "This book is an invitation to come back to the present moment and find peace and joy." I didn't know how I was to find either in my current situation, but I kept reading until I got to the paragraphs on conscious breathing.

> *As you breathe in, you say to yourself, "Breathing in, I know that I am breathing in." And as you breathe out, say, "Breathing out, I know that I am breathing out." Just that. You recognize your in-breath as an in-breath and your out-breath as an out-breath. You don't even need to recite the whole sentence; you can use just two words: "In" and "Out."*

I lay the book on my chest and closed my eyes and took a deep breath. *Breathing in. I know I am breathing in.* Then out. *Breathing out. I know I am breathing out.* I did it again and again, focusing on each breath in and each breath out. And somehow I felt myself settling into my own body. I could feel something—tension, fear?—give way, just a little. Under my closed lids, I could feel the tears, and I let them run down my cheeks, but I didn't stop breathing. I didn't stop noticing my breath. *I'm here. I'm breathing. I'm alive.*

———

On Monday morning, I woke early and showered before waking the boys and starting our morning routine. I tried to put the MRI out of my mind while we got the boys ready for school, but I couldn't. I was scared. But I smiled and tried to keep my voice light as I kissed them goodbye when the bus arrived.

Then Allan drove me to the Nassau Radiologic office. Although I was terrified by what the MRI would reveal, I was also beginning to feel a sense of acceptance take root in me. I knew we would be able to handle whatever lay ahead. We had to.

The technicians agreed to let Allan stay in the room with me during the MRI, which was a relief; I wanted him nearby. They brought in a chair for him, and through the mirror in the tube I could see him leaning on the arm of the chair, a worried expression on his face. If he knew I could see him, he would have tried to keep the frown from his face. But his expression didn't matter; simply his presence helped me relax.

I lay as still as possible in that long tube and thought of my mom and how her calmness in the face of her cancer had calmed *me*. She had glided through the days leading up to her surgery and seemed to have made peace with whatever the outcome would be.

With that awful clanking in my ears, I realized how important my mental outlook would be in the coming days and weeks. I needed to be strong for myself but also for the boys and Allan. I needed to channel my mother's composure, her acceptance. In between the clanking, I took a deep breath, then another one. *Breathe in, Robyn. Breathe out. Breathe in. Breathe out.*

17

THE MRI CONFIRMED what we already knew: cancer, a small lump. But I clung to the word "small" and tried not to imagine the worst. We'd know more after seeing Dr. Kostroff. So until then, I kept busy with the boys, listened to the CDs Ruth gave me, and tried to remember to breathe.

On Wednesday morning, Allan drove me the 15 minutes to Dr. Kostroff's office in New Hyde Park. He dropped me at the door and then parked the car as I made my way into the building and up the elevator to the second floor. I was nervous, but the moment I stepped into her office, I felt myself relax. The waiting area was decorated in soft shades of lavender and sage. Flowers in glass vases lined the receptionist's desk. She smiled when I checked in and gave me a clipboard with forms I needed to complete.

I sat down on one of the comfortable couches and glanced around the room. There were several other women waiting, and I wondered if they, too, had cancer. Or maybe they were survivors. The thought filled me with hope but also gave me the chills. When Allan came in and sat down next to me a few minutes later, I was shaking.

"Are you okay? What's going on?"

"I don't know," I said. "I just started shaking."

Allan put his arm around me and kissed the top of my head. I leaned into him and let his warmth seep into me.

I was still trembling as I filled out the forms, my handwriting shaky. Allan put my coat over my shoulders and rubbed my back, but it felt like the chill had settled in my bones. When I finished with the forms, Allan returned them to the receptionist, and a nurse led us to Dr. Kostroff's office, which was filled with bright sunlight.

Dr. Kostroff was sitting in front of a large window, but when we came in, she stood and shook our hands, smiling warmly. I took a deep breath, knowing I'd made the right choice to see her.

Allan and I sat down across from her, and she listened patiently as I described the last few days, nodding slowly, her eyes kind. Then she asked quietly about my family history of cancer, and I told her about my mom's cancer and that she'd needed surgery and radiation. Even though I knew there were others waiting to see her, Dr. Kostroff made me feel as if I was her only patient.

"Have you had a genetic consultation?"

I nodded. "After my mom's cancer I was tested for the BRCA1 and BRCA2 genes, but the test results were negative."

Dr. Kostroff nodded, brushing her curly light brown hair from her eyes. "That's good news."

Allan squeezed my hand.

"Based on your MRI you'll only need surgery to remove the tumor, most likely followed by radiation. But I can't say definitively. We'll have to see what the pathology report shows." She told us that the morning of my surgery I'd be admitted to Long Island Jewish Hospital. It was the same hospital where I was born and where the boys were born, and this reassured me.

"It's outpatient, so you'll be able to go home the same day."

"What a relief," I said. I explained that the boys had autism and it was hard for me to be away for the night.

"You can go home, but you'll have to take it easy." She smiled, and I nodded, though I knew that wouldn't be easy for me.

Dr. Kostroff reached out and held my hand in hers. "The surgery will go smoothly. Your job now is to go and enjoy your day."

"Thank you so much for getting me in so soon," I said.

"My pleasure."

Allan and I held hands as we left her office. "She was wonderful," Allan said.

I agreed. I knew I'd be getting the best care possible.

The surgery was scheduled for the following Tuesday, and the days until then would be filled with preparation. We still had a few hours before the boys got home from school, and ordinarily Allan and I would have split up to do errands, or we'd have gone home to get some work done. But "ordinary" no longer made sense.

"Let's go out to lunch," I said.

"Really?"

"Yes. Let's just spend the day together."

"I love you," Allan said, unlocking my car door.

"I love you, too," I said, giving him a tight hug before getting into the car.

We drove to the local bagel shop for soup and sandwiches, and as we sat there across from each other, I realized I couldn't remember the last time we'd gone out for lunch, just the two of us.

We were both quieter than usual, and I could feel the weight of the diagnosis and upcoming surgery, but I think we were both relieved to have met Dr. Kostroff, who was even more wonderful than I'd hoped. We ate slowly and then picked up bagels for the boys.

At home, I took care of a few work emails while Allan spread cream cheese on bagels for the boys. Then I programmed Alie's activity schedule, moving the pictures for puzzle and some vocational tasks (card bundling and coin rolling), computer, and piano onto the Velcro strip in his activity notebook even though I knew he'd rush through them.

———

That night after the boys were in bed and I had gotten everything ready for the next day, Allan and I sat on the couch in the den, an itinerary between us as we figured out how to fill the gaps during surgery week and afterward. We didn't yet know how much help we'd need or for how long, but we needed to make sure the boys would be taken care of. Thankfully, all of our home therapists had offered to work extra hours. And our niece, Cheri, had offered to come and stay with us the week after surgery, which was a huge relief because the boys loved her.

Allan had also called Theresa that afternoon to tell her about my diagnosis and the surgery and ask if she would consider coming back to help us with cooking and cleaning for a few weeks after Cheri's visit. She immediately agreed, even though it meant long days for her. But that's how she was. She spent hours each week volunteering at her church and taking meals to congregants in need, somehow finding time for all of that even though she had just opened her own business. I was relieved that she'd be able to help around the house, but I was also looking forward to having her calming presence around us again. We'd missed her over the year since she'd been gone. We all loved her vegetarian cooking, but also her serenity and gentleness.

———

I gathered all of our important papers: our finances, the boys' medical and school records, and the records from our home program. I knew Allan was worried that I might die on the operating table. How would the boys react? What would they do without their mother? How would he handle their care on his own? We both trusted Dr. Kostroff, but sometimes things went wrong. I thought of my mom and the months in the hospital leading up to her death when it was one setback after another. The possibility of my death hung between Allan and me as we sat next to each other, reviewing document after document.

If anything has the power to put your life in perspective, it's cancer. Over the next few days, I felt myself slowing down, noticing things I hadn't noticed before: the thin quality of winter sunlight through the bare branches in the backyard; the brittle crunch of ice under my feet as I walked to the car. Oddly, I felt more alive than ever. I thought of Ruth's words to me on the phone the day of the diagnosis: "You have to put yourself first." And I knew she was right. If there was any time that made sense for me to concentrate on myself, it was now.

After the boys left on the bus in the morning, instead of going into my office to check emails and return phone calls, I bundled up and headed out the door. The cold morning air was unforgiving, but I didn't mind the sting in my lungs. I walked along the icy sidewalk toward the center of town, watching the last of the morning commuters make their way to the train. I smiled at their set faces and their rushing, knowing I usually looked the same way.

I thought of my mom, who had always seemed to put others first—she modeled that for me all those years—but now I realized that she had also taken care of herself, doing the things she loved: spending time with friends; going to the theater; sitting for hours at the library immersed in books, one of her many passions. I knew I would never have that much freedom. The boys wouldn't ever embark on their own lives, leaving Allan and me free to explore untapped interests. I knew we'd always be juggling and tag-teaming and trying to stay ahead of their always changing behaviors. But I needed to figure out how to better take care of myself now, within the confines of the life we were living.

That week, I listened to the meditation CDs that Ruth had loaned me each night before bed. My favorite was *Guided Meditation* by Bodhipaksa, whose soothing voice helped me focus on my body and breathing. As I lay there night after night, I followed my breath, thinking only of that moment, the weight of my body on the bed. When I opened my eyes after 20 minutes, I felt more peaceful than I'd ever felt in my life. I knew I couldn't control the outcome of my surgery or the prognosis, but I could imagine my body free of cancer and I could take care of myself and learn to cultivate tranquility.

———

Saturday was the Snowflake 4 Mile Run in Long Beach, and I was relieved to shift my focus to the boys' running. This was their third year running the Snowflake race so we were familiar with the race setup, which always made things easier. Randy would be running with Jamie, and Kevin with Alie. I was also looking forward to seeing Linda, who had helped us get the boys on the South cross-country team. She was running, as well. And Randy invited us all over for bagels at her condo after the race.

I woke the boys early, starting with Jamie at 5:45 AM. Jamie had become even more resistant to rushing and took more time than ever in the morning to get ready, so I had begun to wake him first to make sure he had the time he needed. Alie, as always, would wake up and rush through each step—anything to get to the starting line quickly. I told them that they'd be running at the beach, and they both smiled. Maybe they recalled the previous years' races. I was always surprised by the things they remembered.

Alie packed the cooler with water and Gatorade, then ate his breakfast as he stared at the cooler and the orange Nike bag, which I had packed with hats, gloves, and extra shirts in case it was windy at the shore, and dry shirts to change into after the race.

It was still dark when we left the house, but soon pale light filled the morning sky. Alie and Jamie stared out their windows and I watched as pink spread across the horizon. "Isn't that beautiful?" I said, and Allan nodded, reaching for my hand.

I was looking forward to being in the chaotic excitement at the starting line, which always gave me a shot of adrenaline. We made our way through the crowds to pick up our bibs, and then we spotted Randy and Linda and Kevin.

Randy gave me a hug. "You look great! You're going to beat this thing."

"I have to," I said.

"You will," Randy said. "I know it."

At the starting line, Kevin and Alie lined up in the front, Jamie and Randy in the middle of the pack, and Linda close behind them. There were about 500 people running that day, and as we stood there in the crowd, I thought about what an important part of our lives this had become: practices, races, the camaraderie at the starting line. I wanted to be around for all of the boys' races, always.

Allan and I moved to the side and rubbed our hands together as we waited for the runners to loop back down the boardwalk. "Do you wish you were running?"

"Kind of," Allan said. "But I'm not sure I'm ready for four miles yet. And I'd rather be here with you." He put his arm around me, and I leaned into him.

The boys had a great race. Alie ran it in 27:57, a seven-minute pace, and Jamie did it in 35:37, an 8:55 pace. Both of them were beaming as they came barreling down the boardwalk. Later we all met back at Randy's condo, where she set out bagels, cream cheese, and lox, and I unwrapped the fruit platter we'd brought.

We filled the boys' plates with food, and they seemed content to sit with everyone as we chatted and ate, though I had to watch Alie closely so he wouldn't eat too much too fast and choke or throw up.

I was relieved that no one brought up my surgery, happy instead to listen to Randy and Kevin and Linda and Allan talk running and upcoming races. Allan hoped to run his first race with Jamie that winter or spring, but we weren't sure what we'd be able to commit to now. We'd just have to wait and see.

————

Three days later on Tuesday morning, I woke up feeling calm. I went into the bathroom and turned on the shower and slowly undressed as steam filled the room. I stepped into the stream of hot water and wondered how my body would be changed after today. I was anxious to get the tumor out of me, but I wondered how I'd feel about my body afterward. Would I have a bad scar?

The night before, as we climbed into bed, Allan told me that he loved me and said how beautiful I was. Over the years he must have told me that thousands of times, and perhaps I'd taken it for granted, but I didn't take it for granted now. As we held each other, he whispered, "And you'll be beautiful always, no matter what."

But I didn't feel beautiful as I stared at myself in the mirror, drying my hair. I looked tired, raw, somehow older. I knew I wasn't supposed to wear any makeup, but I didn't want to go into surgery looking the way I did. I wanted to look alive. So I put on a little mascara and just a little lipstick. They weren't operating on my face, after all. I nodded at the result before going in to wake Jamie and Alie.

That morning, I hugged and kissed the boys, wishing I could somehow slow everything down, suspend us all in time. But of course I couldn't. When the bus arrived, I hugged Alie tightly. "I love you."

Alie said, "ah o ooh," his version of "I love you," and then he rushed through the open door of the bus.

Then I hugged Jamie and told him I loved him.

"Ah lova you," Jamie said. Then he looked down at the laces on his sneakers and bent down to fix the loops so that they were the exact same size.

I waved as the bus pulled away from the curb.

Allan and I were quiet on the drive to the hospital. I could tell he was nervous, but I didn't feel scared. I knew surgery was just the first step, and the journey we were suddenly on might be a long one, but I felt ready. I focused on taking breaths into my belly, imagining light filling me up.

Lakeville Road was bumper-to-bumper traffic, and normally I'd be irritated by the delay. But today I wasn't; we had plenty of time to get to the hospital. I stared out the window at the bare winter trees that lined the street. Soon they would begin to bud, and the earliest spring flowers would begin to push their way through the thawing ground. I would be around to see it happen. The surgery would go well, without a hitch. I had to believe that.

When we got to Long Island Jewish Hospital, Allan dropped me at the entrance and went to park the car while I walked to the ambulatory surgical center. I checked in and sat down to wait for Allan. I felt at peace. I knew I had prepared myself as best as I could for the day, and I felt a sense of tranquility.

When Allan joined me in the waiting room, he tilted his head and looked at me with a quizzical expression. "You look so calm."

"I know, I feel good."

"I'm just surprised by how calm you are." He shook his head. "You're going into freakin' surgery, and I've never seen you so calm. It's eerie."

I smiled. It was as if I had been flooded with positive energy. I couldn't explain it, but I knew it would take me through the next few hours. I imagined being well, whole.

A few minutes later, a nurse called my name, and Allan and I were led to a large room with curtained cubicles where I would be prepped for surgery. Men and women, some wearing hospital gowns, some wearing regular clothes, sat on light blue vinyl recliners, surrounded by family or friends. I was asked to verify who I was, my date of birth, and my address before a wristband was tightened on my wrist. *This is really happening*, I thought. *But I'm ready.*

Then the nurse handed me a gown and closed the curtain. I changed and then she came back to take my vitals and insert an IV.

"I just can't believe how calm you are," Allan said again.

In that moment I realized that all of this was probably harder for him than it was for me. Poor Allan, he looked so pale. I smiled. "I'm going to be fine."

Just then the anesthesiologist came in, followed by Dr. Kostroff. I was actually more nervous about the anesthesia than I was about the surgery. I hated being sedated, hated the thought of relinquishing control like that. But I knew I just had to give into it. Let go.

"How are you feeling?" Dr. Kostroff asked.

"Okay," I said. "Fine, actually."

She nodded.

"Do you have any questions?" the anesthesiologist asked, but I shook my head.

"Okay then," he said. "We'll be starting in a few minutes. We're a team here and we'll take good care of you."

When the nurse came back a few minutes later to take me to the operating room, Allan leaned over and kissed me, forcing a smile. "I love you," he said, his voice shaky.

"I love you too," I said. "Take care of the boys."

Then I walked through the doors to the operating room.

18

When I woke up in the recovery room Allan was standing at the foot of the bed.

"Hi," I said quietly.

He smiled. "The doctor says it went well."

Dr. Kostroff came in then. She was still wearing scrubs, her hair tucked under a surgical cap. I almost didn't recognize her. "The surgery went perfectly," she said, taking my hand in hers. "You did great, and we only had to take out the tumor. The lymph nodes were all negative."

"Thank God," I said, feeling myself relax.

My orders were to rest. I was exhausted, so that sounded like an easy request. The boys were covered by our home therapists, and our niece, Cheri, would be arriving that day to help, as well. She lived in Minnesota near the rest of Allan's family but was spending a year in Provincetown, Massachusetts as a writing fellow at the Fine Arts Works Center. I was relieved she'd be there because she was full of bubbly energy.

Everything was in order and the surgery had gone well. As Allan helped me out of the car an hour later, I was sore but elated.

————

Over the next few days, I tried not to worry about the pathology report, which I'd get the following Monday at my post-op appointment with Dr. Kostroff. Having Cheri around helped keep my mind off it. Her laughter was contagious, and Jamie, especially, loved to snuggle up to her on the couch. While the boys were at school, Cheri and Allan and

I watched movies together, which felt decadent—a movie during the day!—and Cheri cooked, one day making a delicious tortellini with sun dried tomatoes and fresh mozzarella. On Valentine's Day, two days after my surgery, Cheri and Allan went out shopping and returned with a Valentine's cupcake for me and coloring books for the boys.

I spent hours resting and reading my self-healing and meditation books while Cheri colored and read books with the boys. I felt strong, and after a couple of days no longer needed Tylenol. My incision didn't really bother me. It was covered with gauze and bandages so I couldn't see how large the wound was, but based on what Dr. Kostroff said, it was small.

After a few days, Cheri headed back to Provincetown, and though I continued to take things slow, I was ready for the next step, ready to beat the cancer.

The following Monday, Allan and I drove back to Dr. Kostroff's office. We were ushered into her sunny office once again and sat down across from her.

"Well," she said, "as I suspected based on the size of your tumor, which was 0.5 cm, you have early-stage cancer. That's good news." She paused and smiled. "But the pathology showed that it was HER2-positive."

I reached for Allan's hand. I didn't know what that meant, but I could tell it wasn't good.

"What's HER2-positive?"

She explained that HER2 was a protein that stimulated growth in breast cancer cells and that HER2-positive meant I had a more aggressive form of cancer. I felt like I'd been punched in the stomach. All of the hope I'd nurtured the previous week vanished.

"The good news is that we now have targeted therapy for HER2-positive tumors," Dr. Kostroff said softly. I knew she could tell that Allan and I were scared, and she was trying to do her best to reassure us. "It's called Herceptin, and it attaches itself to the HER2 receptors and blocks growth signals."

Dr. Kostroff reached across the table for my free hand, which was trembling. "Herceptin is fairly new, but it's very promising. Early-stage breast cancer patients with HER2-positive tumors one centimeter or smaller are at significant risk of recurrence of their disease, but Herceptin has also reduced the risk of recurrence."

"So what does this mean?" Allan asked.

"You will need radiation for certain and most likely Herceptin, but because you're HER2-positive you may also need additional treatment."

"Treatment?" I was confused.

"Chemotherapy," she said.

At the mention of chemo, I went cold. Years earlier I had been diagnosed with neutropenia, an abnormally low level of neutrophils, a type of white blood cell. And I knew that chemotherapy could dangerously compromise my immune system by lowering my white blood cell count even more. I thought of Allan's boss from the real estate firm, who had died after her body was ravaged by chemo. The same thing happened to my uncle Gerry, my mom's brother. Their bodies couldn't withstand the effects of the chemo, and their immune systems just broke down.

Dr. Kostroff picked up the phone and scheduled an appointment for me with an oncologist for the following week. Then she took my hand in hers again. "We caught it early, which is good. But the oncologist will have a better sense of the appropriate course of treatment."

I nodded, my eyes full of tears. She was so reassuring that I hated to leave her office and go home, where Allan and I would have to face this new reality on our own. I felt blindsided, not having really entertained the fact that I might need chemo. But Dr. Kostroff only said that it was a possibility. Maybe I wouldn't need it at all.

We were quiet on the short drive home. I stared out the window at the slushy streets, the cloudy sky oppressive. We passed Long

Island Jewish Hospital, and I imagined the people in the oncology unit, fighting cancers much more advanced than mine. I gave myself a mental shake. Be grateful we caught it so early. But I couldn't dispel the fear that had lodged itself like a sliver in my heart. Chemo. What would this mean for me?

When we got home, Allan and I collapsed on the couch. We hugged each other tightly, both of us numb. I couldn't even begin to make sense of it all: aggressive cancer, high rate of recurrence, all those drugs.

"We just have to wait and see what the oncologist says," Allan said, forcing a smile.

I nodded. "I know."

———

Theresa began working for us again that afternoon, and I was so grateful not to have to worry about cooking and laundry. She gave me a hug when she arrived and then made herself at home in the kitchen. On the phone I'd told her that my naturopath had suggested eliminating dairy, soy, caffeine, alcohol, and sugar from my diet, and Theresa, who only cooked organic vegetarian food, was determined that I would follow each and every one of Dr. Stills' recommendations. That day she brought pounds of raw almonds with her and made homemade almond milk for me and brewed some immune-boosting tea, determined to cure me.

I sat in the den, dull gray light seeping through the windows, trying not to worry as I waited for the boys to come home. Theresa came in and handed me a cup of tea, and tears filled my eyes. I was so grateful to have so many loving, caring people in my life. I wondered if I deserved them. Over the years I had so often been exhausted or crabby, wrapped up in my self-absorbed routine. Had I been a good friend? I hoped so. My friends were there for me, again and again, always.

———

Allan and I assumed that I'd meet with the oncologist and have a plan in place within a week. I wanted to get started with whatever treatment was recommended so that I could put it all behind me and get on with my life. But things didn't go as smoothly as we had expected. The first oncologist I saw recommended a cocktail of chemo drugs, Herceptin, and radiation, followed by an aromatase inhibitor (AI) for five years to lower my estrogen levels and reduce the risk of recurrence. I hadn't expected I'd need such aggressive treatment, and I was devastated. We asked about my neutropenia and how that would be affected by the chemo, and he said that I would need weekly shots of Neupogen to stimulate my white blood cell growth. Months later, I would wish that we had taken this doctor's recommendation and had gotten started right away with the treatment, but Allan and I were both so overwhelmed and scared by how chemo would affect my immune system that we wanted to make sure it was really necessary.

So I sought a second opinion, and that doctor's recommendation was only radiation and an AI. He wasn't convinced I needed Herceptin. Herceptin without chemo wasn't the protocol, so its recommended use varied from doctor to doctor. We were relieved, especially because we learned that Herceptin would also affect my white blood count. But because the opinions were so drastically different, I made an appointment with a third oncologist.

His recommendation was similar to that of the first oncologist: radiation, AI, Herceptin, and maybe chemo, though he was hesitant about adding the chemo because of my low white blood count.

Because my tumor was 0.5 cm, that put it in a gray area in terms of the recommended course of action. In 2008, if a tumor was smaller than 1 cm, chemo was often not recommended. But because my tumor was HER2-positive, that complicated things.

I was reeling, unsure whom to trust. The lack of consensus about whether or not I needed chemo or even Herceptin made me feel panicked. So I consulted a fourth doctor, and she recommended just Herceptin and radiation, followed by an AI. We were once again relieved and we decided, finally, to go with her recommendation. But the next day she called to say that with more thought she decided to add the chemo to her initial course of treatment. Then a few days later, she changed it back again: just radiation, Herceptin, and an AI. She was leaving for vacation but told us she was now convinced that I wouldn't need chemo and that I could start the Herceptin when she returned.

I decided to put the chemo out of my mind, focusing on the other tests I needed to get before I could begin the Herceptin infusions. We learned that in addition to causing flu-like symptoms in 40 percent of patients, Herceptin could affect how well the heart pumps blood and in some cases lead to congestive heart failure, heart attack, and even death. But there was no question about not taking Herceptin; the more research I did on the HER2 protein, the more convinced I was that Herceptin was a must. So I scheduled an appointment with Dr. Gupta, my internist, for a baseline echocardiogram.

I spent the rest of the week working and eating well and trying to get plenty of rest. Each night before bed, I listened to my meditation CD, and I felt good, calm. We had bumped the boys up to running three days a week, so on Tuesday and Thursday afternoons and Saturday mornings, Allan and I drove Alie and Jamie out to Bethpage State Park to meet Kevin. While they ran, I walked slowly along the bike path, grateful for the sun on my back.

———

Allan was on his own mission to make sure I did everything I could do to take care of myself and beat the cancer. He scoured the Internet and paged through stacks of natural healing books. Every morning he made me my immune-booster smoothie, and he began to leave articles plastered with Post-it notes around the house: "Read this."

One of the articles described how moderate exercise three to five times a week could "reduce the risk of breast cancer by 30–40 percent." But since I already had cancer, that wasn't too helpful. But another article cited the effects that physical activity had on hormones and energy balance and described the correlation between exercise and survival rates in breast cancer patients, stating that women with cancer who exercised moderately five hours a week reduced their risk of dying of a breast cancer related death by more than half. More than half.

That afternoon before the boys got home, Allan asked whether I'd read the articles.

"I did," I said, knowing that I was about to get a lecture.

"You have to start exercising," he said, leaning against the counter in the kitchen, staring at me as if he expected a battle. "It's a no brainer! You can join a gym and start taking aerobics classes again."

But though I'd loved aerobics before the boys were born, the thought of jumping and lunging in a room crowded with other people no longer appealed to me at all. Not to mention the fact that all that quick movement would likely exacerbate my vertigo.

"I'll see," I said, taking a sip of my tea. "Let's just see how the Herceptin and radiation affect me."

But Allan wasn't going to let it go. "You can't say no to this," he said, glaring at me. "Rob, you're a control freak. This is something that you can control. You have to start exercising and you have to commit to it."

"I walk and bike sometimes," I said.

Allan shook his head. "You don't do it consistently. You need to commit to it."

"Fine," I said, irritated. "But can you give me a break for now?"

"I think you should start running," he said. "Look at what its done for me."

It was true that Allan hadn't felt this good in years. He had clearly gained strength and flexibility in the months since he'd started running, and he'd lost a little weight. He was still overcome by intense fatigue in the afternoons and he still tripped and frequently fell on runs, but he swore it was worth it.

"I don't know," I said. Running had been all about the boys and more recently about the boys and Allan. I had never been interested in lacing up my own shoes. And I certainly couldn't imagine starting to run right now before my treatment and after all the indecision of the last few weeks.

Allan threw his hands in the air. "I need you to promise me you'll try it. The boys need you."

He knew that mentioning the boys would hit a nerve, and it did. I felt a spark of anger. Of course I'd do anything in my control to increase my chances of survival for the sake of Alie and Jamie. He knew that.

"Promise me you'll try it," Allan said, his voice softer now.

"Of course," I said quietly. "I will. Soon."

When he continued to glare at me, I added, "I promise."

———

The following week, when we went to meet with the oncologist to outline the schedule for the radiation and Herceptin, she told us that she had changed her mind once again and decided that I should have chemo after all. I could feel Allan seething next to me, but I didn't even have the energy to get angry. I felt utterly exhausted.

"Are you kidding me?" Allan said. "All of this back and forth is totally unacceptable!"

She said she had consulted with colleagues and decided, now definitively, that I needed the chemo.

Allan clenched his jaw. "You have no idea how much stress you've caused us with your indecision!"

Later, he was still furious about her waffling. "It's outrageous."

I agreed, but if I really needed the chemo, I couldn't put it off any longer. We didn't have time to find a new doctor. All of the back and forth had delayed the start of my treatment, and I still wasn't sure we were even doing the right thing.

That afternoon I called Dr. Kostroff, explaining the different opinions and asking for her help. "Oh Robyn, I'm sorry," she said. "I know how stressful this has been." Then she suggested that she present my case to the Oncology Tumor Board, consisting of the top oncologists in the area.

"Yes! Please!" I said, flooded with relief.

A few days later, my case was presented to the Tumor Board and Dr. Kostroff called with the unanimous decision to treat my cancer with the chemo drug Taxol, Herceptin, and radiation. I would need weekly chemo for 12 weeks, followed by radiation five days a week for five weeks. I'd get the weekly Herceptin infusions for a full year and then begin a five-year daily dose of an AI.

"I know this is not what you'd hoped to hear," she said, her voice gentle. "But they all agreed that treating it aggressively was the best approach. And you need to start right away."

I felt defeated but also, finally, relieved that there was a definitive decision. I began researching Taxol and its side effects, which ranged from fatigue and nausea to numbness in the hands and feet to decreased liver function. But I resigned myself to the risks. I went to see Dr. Stills, who didn't want me to go through with the chemo, but she supported my decision and gave me lists of herbs and supplements that would help my body detox.

Because the board recommended I start chemo right away, I'd have to do so under the supervision of the most recent oncologist, who had switched her mind four times. But neither Allan nor I wanted her to be responsible for my ongoing care, so I asked Dr. Kostroff for another recommendation. She put us in touch with Dr. Vincent Vinciguerra, and I scheduled an appointment for the following week.

———

A few days later, Allan drove me to my first chemo treatment. We checked in and walked into the treatment room, which was crowded with other patients, all getting infusions. I was shown to one of the leather chairs, and as I sat down I glanced around the room. The other patients all looked sick, some of them very sick. Some were bald and others not, and I wondered if they were wearing wigs. I couldn't imagine losing my hair, though I knew it would happen. Allan glanced around the room, as well, and I could tell he was uncomfortable, shifting from foot to foot.

A few days earlier I'd been given a shot of Neupogen to increase my white blood count, and it had worked, increasing it enough for me to withstand the chemo. So now the nurse inserted an IV into the top of my right hand, then she smiled and laid a blanket across my lap. "You might feel cold," she said, and I nodded, unfolding it and spreading it over my legs.

I held a list of the infusion drugs I was being given and a photograph of Alie and Jamie at age 13, grinning in front of an Italian café at Disney World. Allan stood next to me, his brow furrowed. I knew he was scared but also that he didn't approve. I, too, couldn't believe that I was voluntarily accepting all of that poison into my body. But I was going to do whatever would give me the best chance of survival. I stared up at the IV stand, at the bright orange and clear bags waiting to be pumped into me, and felt my stomach clench. But I knew I had to be strong. I had to get through this so I could be there for the boys.

I suddenly felt dizzy. I took a deep breath, then another. I wanted to fill myself with light, with warmth. *I'm grateful for my family. I'm grateful for my friends. I'm grateful for my boys.* I looked down at the photo of Alie and Jamie, at their smiling faces.

"We're going to beat this," Allan said, and squeezed my hand.

Suddenly I felt the cold rush of liquid snaking through my veins—*Breathe, Robyn, Breathe*—and then another wave of dizziness that forced me to close my eyes. Each time I began to wonder what would happen to the boys if I didn't make it, I'd try to release those thoughts, let them go. I leaned my head back against the leather chair and took breath after breath, trying to focus on what I *could* control. *I can take deep breaths. I can eat well. I can exercise. I'll be strong. I'll be strong.*

The infusion took almost two hours, and by the time it was done, I was exhausted and light-headed and couldn't wait to get home to sleep. I closed my eyes on the way home and then went straight to bed, sleeping for three hours.

That afternoon, my friend Brenda arrived to stay for two nights. I'd known Brenda since we were teenagers, and though she and her husband lived in Connecticut and we didn't see one another very often, we were still very close and talked regularly on the phone. I knew she'd keep things light and keep me laughing, which she did. That first night we reminisced about high school and our wild teenage years. But as we were talking, I would start a sentence and then completely forget the next word. My mind just went blank. Both she and Allan stared at me waiting for the words to emerge, but I couldn't coax them out. "Chemo brain," I joked, having read about the memory loss and fogginess that could accompany chemo, and we laughed it off even though it was disconcerting to not be able to think straight.

After Brenda left, I began working a little from home. Though I'd felt wiped out for a couple of days after that first infusion, as the week wore on, I started to feel better. And I realized that it was time to follow through on my promise to Allan.

So the following week, three days after my second chemo session, I decided it was time to start running. It was the beginning of April, and as I opened the door and stepped out into the bright sun,

I took a deep breath, filling my lungs with cold, fresh air. I zipped up my jacket and started to run, one foot in front of the other, down the hill and around the bend. *I'm going to beat this*, I thought. *I'm strong.*

I was slow and was out of breath by the end of the block. How could the boys and Allan run as far and fast as they did? I couldn't imagine it. But I knew I was doing the right thing. I ran down the hill at the end of our block, taking in the green of the budding trees. In our neighbors' gardens, bright yellow daffodils and red and pink tulips reached toward the sun. I listened to my footfalls on concrete, and with each step, I felt myself running away from that cold leather chair and the IV bags of bright orange fluid. Instead I was running toward strength, toward wellness.

19

THERE WAS SOMETHING about running—the crisp air, the ache in my lungs—that made me feel alive. It didn't matter that I often struggled to catch my breath. Within a few weeks, running had become my talisman, my rabbit's foot, my good luck charm. I couldn't run for the first few days after each treatment because I was too tired and weak. But by the third day, I felt better, so I would lace up my shoes and head out the door.

After that first run on my own, I began to join the boys and Kevin and Allan when they went out to train. I wasn't fit enough to run with Allan and Jamie yet, so I took off on my own, following the trail into the woods. I would breathe deeply, marveling at the boggy smell of spring, the crunching of old leaves under my feet, the blue sky above me. I used to love watching the boys and Kevin and Allan take off for their practice runs and return intoxicated with the fresh air and exercise, but it was something else to head out by myself and meet them back at the car just as energized as they were.

Allan had slowly increased his miles, and practices with Jamie continued to go well, so he finally felt ready to run his first race with Jamie. We settled on the Jigsaw 4 Mile Run in East Islip. It was a race hosted by the EJ Autism Foundation, which funded Long Island programs for children on the spectrum, so we were happy to participate and support their work.

It was mid-April and a beautiful morning to run: 50 degrees and sunny. This was the boys' first race in two months, and I think we were all craving the excitement and energy of a race day. When we arrived, there were already a ton of runners there, including some Rolling Thunder athletes, warming up and stretching in small groups. Kevin was well-known and well-respected in the Long Island running community, and he was making the rounds, walking from group to group, chatting it up. He was completely in his element, and it was obvious how happy he was.

The Jigsaw course was flat and fast. It started at the marina, wound through the streets of East Islip, along the edge of the inlet, and finished again at the marina. Allan and the boys and I walked across the beach to the registration table where Gina, one of our first therapists who now worked for the EJ Autism Foundation, was handing out bibs and t-shirts. She squealed when she saw us and jumped up to give us hugs. "Alie! Jamie! Hi!"

The boys smiled at her, and she said she couldn't believe what handsome young men they'd become. "And I've heard they're amazing runners." It was hard to imagine them as the twirling, flapping, jumping tornadoes they were when Gina first met them. I stared at the boys, seeing them through Gina's eyes—handsome young athletes—and I felt a wave of pride. They'd come so far. Look at all they'd accomplished. And more importantly, look how happy they were!

Soon, though, they both started bouncing, and I knew they were getting impatient. We gave Gina quick hugs and made our way toward the starting line.

"Are you excited?" I asked Allan.

He nodded, smiling. "It just feels right, doesn't it?"

It did, one of the only "right" things in a long time.

I kissed the boys and Allan, then Kevin took Alie's hand and moved him to the front of the pack, and Allan led Jamie into the middle. As I stood there in the morning chill, surrounded by all those runners waiting for the gun to go off, I thought about how running had been all about the boys and more recently about the boys and Allan. But now I wondered what it would feel like to run my own race.

———

Everyone had a great race. Alie and Kevin ran a 7:01 pace, and Jamie and Allan ran a 10:00 pace, over a minute slower than Jamie's usual time, but he didn't care. He was beaming when he crossed the finish line, and at the post-race celebration he was smiling and jumping, jumping, jumping. "He could have run forever," Allan said.

"How do you feel?" I asked.

"Exhausted!" Allan laughed. "But amazing. Jamie was so happy the whole race. We just fell into a rhythm."

I imagined them looping through the streets of East Islip, not speaking but bound to each other by the sound of their footfalls on the road. And I knew that Allan had been right about running with Jamie. I handed Allan his sweatshirt and gave him a hug.

Both boys were relaxed and smiling for the rest of the day. We all loved the running community and excitement of a race day, and as soon as the boys had run one race, we'd begin planning for the next one.

———

Six months before the East Islip race and well before my cancer diagnosis, Randy and I had talked about hosting a race to benefit Genesis. "I could combine my two loves, autism and running," she said, "*and* benefit Genesis!" We laughed about how fun that would be, but we weren't really serious about it. Undertaking that kind of project would be a huge amount of work. But it kept coming up in conversation— we should host a race!—and one day we just decided to do it.

"Are you serious?" Randy said.

"Yeah, let's do it," I said. We could design a race that raised money for the boys' school *and* highlight the power of running for people with autism. How could we not do it?

We decided that I would be the race director, and we contacted Mike Polansky, the president of the Greater Long Island Running Club (GLIRC), for advice. Mike was excited about it, as well, and we decided to contract with GLIRC to do the race management, which would include measuring the course and taking care of the registration, photos, brochures, promotion, and mailing.

That would leave Randy and me in charge of the name of the race, the venue and food, securing sponsors, designing the logo, and deciding on the awards and giveaways. It was a lot to tackle, but we were committed. And we were joined by our friend Nancy, who was a behavior specialist at Genesis.

Mike suggested a few possible venues where we might stage the race, one of them the Great Neck School District. I loved the idea of holding the race in the boys' home district, so we set up a meeting with the superintendent, Ron Friedman. Ron, who was also a runner, was thrilled about the prospect of partnering with us. He went right over to his computer and pulled up a course map on the campus at Great Neck South, where the boys had run cross-country. It was perfect. And Nancy's daughter Samantha, a student at Great Neck South, agreed to rally the South students to get them involved.

We were already in the thick of planning by the time I was diagnosed with breast cancer. We decided that it would be a four-mile race, Blazing Trails 4-Autism, a name Allan and our niece Cheri came up with, and I had already begun reaching out to potential sponsors. There was no way I was going to cancel it because of the cancer. Besides, planning it filled me with hope in those dark weeks of indecision between my surgery and the beginning of my treatment. And as the year progressed, it would keep me focused on the future, on wellness.

The race was scheduled for November 9. By that point I'd be finished with both the chemo and radiation and I'd be over halfway done with my weekly Herceptin infusions.

I had resigned myself to the weekly chemo, though I hated the sterile, crowded room where I got my infusions. But I knew I'd only be there another week. I had begun the process of shifting my care to my new oncologist, Dr. Vincent Vinciguerra, whom Dr. Kostroff had recommended. He was Chief of the Don Monti Division of Oncology/Hematology at the Monter Cancer Center, part of the North Shore LIJ Health System, across the street from Long Island Jewish Hospital where I'd had my surgery. When Allan and I went for my first appointment with him, I was immediately calmed by the open airiness of the lobby. It was filled with bright sunlight, pine benches, and bamboo trees. And Dr. Vinciguerra was gentle and soft-spoken and concurred with the Tumor Board's treatment decision. Both Allan and I were relieved that I'd finish my treatment under his care.

But in the meantime, I had completed my third infusion and I knew I would begin losing my hair soon, which I dreaded. I had attended a class for breast cancer patients on looking and feeling your best. Ruth went with me as moral support, and I was so glad she was there because I felt strangely nervous when I walked into that room full of bald women. I should have been reassured by the laughter that exploded across the room, but mostly I just felt depressed. I loved my hair, which over the years I had straightened and lightened. Now I couldn't imagine myself without my long blond hair. But there were cosmetologists there to give wig and makeup presentations, and they offered tips to help us feel pretty despite the ravages of chemo. I left feeling that I could still look like myself even without my hair.

I heard about a Hasidic wig designer in town who made wigs of natural hair, so I went to see him and showed him my hair and left pictures with him. I was relieved when he said it wouldn't be a problem to make a natural-looking wig for me.

Then I went to the salon where I'd been going for years. I couldn't bear to have my head completely shaved, but my stylist, Marlene, thought I'd look great with a pixie cut. I wasn't sure about that, but I didn't have a choice, so I nodded and then closed my eyes so I wouldn't have to watch the long chunks of blond hair fall to the floor around me.

When I opened my eyes, I stared into the mirror and hardly recognized myself. Everyone in the salon gathered around and said I looked wonderful, but I didn't see it. I looked like a stranger.

Allan had always loved my long hair, so it surprised me when I got home and he said how much he liked it short. I wasn't sure if he really meant that or if he was just trying to make me feel better. Regardless, I did feel a little better, and I decided that I wouldn't cover it when I was at home. But when I went out, I put on my wig, which thankfully was almost indistinguishable from my real hair.

The pixie didn't last long, anyway. That week, clumps of hair started to fall out in the shower. It was so odd to pull my hands away from my shampooed head only to have them covered in hair. And my scalp felt tender and raw. The one thing that made me feel better was the fact that the chemo had made my hair dry and lifeless anyway. When it started to fall out, it felt like I was getting rid of that poison. But still, when I looked at myself in the mirror without my wig, I looked old and sick.

I had my first treatment at the Monter Cancer Center under Dr. Vinciguerra's care at the beginning of May, and it was a completely different experience. In the treatment room, each patient had their own large cubicle with a television and DVD player and a chair for a visitor. It was private and comfortable, and I was so relieved to have made the change. Before each treatment, I went to the lab there to have my white count checked to make sure the Neupogen shot was still working, which thankfully it was. And during my treatment, Dr. Vinciguerra always came to check on me. I had started experiencing some other unpleasant side effects of the chemo: I was shaky, had nosebleeds, and had developed sores in my mouth. But Dr. Vinciguerra assured me that these would resolve, and I nodded, grateful for his kind manner. I knew that under his care, I'd get better.

———

Later that month, we registered the boys for the Runday 5K in Hicksville, which they'd run the year before. Alie was running with Kevin, as usual. But though Allan had had a good race with Jamie in April, he had been having leg pain and his usual fatigue, and he didn't want to overdo it, so that day Jamie would run with Ray.

Both boys seemed relaxed and excited for the race. Because they'd run it the previous year, they were familiar with the course through the streets of Hicksville and Bethpage. Alie took second in his age group, coming in at 20:26. Then he and Kevin met us near the finish to cheer Jamie on. But when Jamie appeared with Ray, the front of his legs were covered in blood, from his knees all the way to his ankles.

"Oh my God," I said, my stomach dropping. "What the hell happened?"

"Did he fall?" Allan asked, worried. "Or did he get upset?"

"Oh no," Kevin said.

Jamie was still running, but he appeared stressed, his brow furrowed as he ran past us. Allan and I rushed to the finish, where we found Jamie and Ray, who was kneeling down to look at Jamie's knees.

"What happened?" I asked, trying to keep my voice light. I didn't want to further upset Jamie.

Ray shook his head. "He seemed fine, and then all of a sudden, with about a mile left, he yelled and grabbed my arm, and then he just went down," Ray said, and I knew he felt awful. "I helped him up and asked him if he was okay, and he said yes, and then he just started running again."

I put my arm around Jamie's waist. "I'll go get him cleaned up," I said, leading him through the crowd to the first aid tent.

When the volunteer saw Jamie's knees, she said, "What happened?"

I grimaced. "I'm not sure. He has autism and can't tell me. But I think he was upset and just threw himself down."

"Yikes," she said. "Do you want me to take a look?"

"I can do it," I said. She nodded and handed me towels and water, peroxide, and bandages.

"Sit here, Jamie," I said, patting the chair, then I knelt down in front of him. I was trying to stay calm, but I felt like crying as I wiped the blood from his legs and, as gently as I could, picked the gravel from his kneecaps. It broke my heart that he couldn't even tell me what happened or how he felt.

It reminded me of when he was eight and seemed to be coming down with a cold. He was lethargic, not bouncing around as he usually did, and he had a slight fever. He wasn't coughing or sneezing, though, so I thought I'd wait a day or two and see if he improved. But he didn't get better; he just looked at me with sad eyes, unable to say if he felt nauseated or if anything hurt. After a couple of days I took him to the doctor, who took one look at him and told us to go straight to the ER.

I was horrified. It turned out he had pneumonia and was seriously dehydrated, so they had to hook him up to IV antibiotics and fluids. I had watched him so closely, trying to figure out what was wrong, but in the end I missed it because he couldn't tell me how he felt. He must have been miserable and was probably delirious from dehydration because as he lay on the hospital bed, he reached out his hand and said "help me," something he'd never done before.

Now, I gently cleaned Jamie's knees with peroxide and applied an antibiotic ointment to the cuts, covering them with bandages. I hated that he couldn't tell me what had upset him on the run.

"Are you okay now?" I asked quietly.

"Yessss," he said. And he did seem okay. Even though his knees must have hurt, they didn't seem to bother him. He smiled then, as if to say he was sorry, or maybe that he was ready to go back out and join the post-race celebration.

"Okay," I said, making my voice light and chipper. "Let's go and have some fun."

But Allan and I both felt heavy as we left Hicksville. "I feel so guilty," he said in the car on the way home. "I wish I had been running with him today. Maybe this wouldn't have happened."

"I know," I said, thinking the same thing. "But you can't run every race."

"Well, I'll have to." He pursed his lips. "That can't happen again."

I agreed, but I also didn't want Allan to push himself.

"I'm getting stronger and stronger. I can do this."

———

I, too, was getting stronger despite my weekly infusions of chemo and Herceptin. I had joined 30 Minute Fitness, a gym in Great Neck, and had been working with a personal trainer weekly, lifting weights and strengthening my core. Each week I felt healthier, more athletic and more grounded emotionally. I wondered why it had taken me all these years to take care of myself. Certainly I had been busy, especially when I was working full time, but now I realized I could have carved out time for myself. I was determined to do it from now on.

I started to run with Allan and Jamie when they trained. Jamie seemed to like having me there, running along with them, though I often trailed behind. He'd periodically look back, as if checking to make sure I was still there. I'd wave and yell, "I'm here. Keep going!" On hot days, though, I'd bike rather than run because running made me overheat. I wasn't sure if it was the chemo, but I could no longer tolerate the heat, often feeling lightheaded.

The cumulative effects of the chemo were making me more and more tired, but I wanted to do something big to celebrate the boys on their golden birthday, June 18. So after talking with Allan, we decided to host a birthday party for them at Genesis. I rented tents and ordered pizza and balloons. Joe, the boys' therapist, agreed to act as DJ, which I knew all the kids would love. We invited the whole school program: staff and students as well as the Great Neck transportation staff, who got the boys to and from school each day. My dad would have loved it. I could almost picture him there, throwing his head back and laughing as he watched all the festivities.

I was completely bald at this point and was wearing my wig, but it was a humid day, and I could feel my scalp sweating. But it didn't matter. There were hugs and high fives, and Alie and Jamie stood smiling and bouncing to the music. I only had one more chemo infusion ahead of me, and the party felt like a celebration of not only their lives and my life as their mother but also of our future together.

On Monday, June 23, I drove myself to my last chemo treatment. I was so relieved that the Neupogen shot had been effective and that my white blood count had held up. All the nurses knew it was my last chemo infusion and they greeted me with smiles. I'd be back weekly for the infusions of Herceptin, of course, but getting through chemo was something to celebrate.

As I leaned back in the chair waiting for that now-familiar wave of dizziness, I thought of the summer ahead: the races, my weekly visits to the gym, runs with the boys and Allan. I knew behaviors would pop up for the boys as they always did, but none of that mattered in that moment. We would take care of those as they cropped up, and I'd be grateful for each day.

20

THAT SUMMER WAS FILLED with training and races, preparation for the Blazing Trails race, and radiation. It was decided that I'd need at least six weeks of radiation, five days a week. Back in March I had had my first appointment with a radiologist at Long Island Radiology and had gotten the tattoos marking the treatment field, which ensured that the radiation angles would accurately target the correct spot on my breast while avoiding grazing my heart.

Compared to the chemo, radiation was quick and easy. My first session was on July 15, and I was calm as I lay down on the table in the radiation treatment room. As instructed, I held as still as possible as the red laser-like light was aimed at my breast. It was the kind of laser you'd see in a spy movie, the hero jumping over and sliding under it, careful to avoid tripping a silent alarm. But there was no escaping this laser, and of course I didn't want to. Everything had been carefully calibrated so that beam of light would kill any remaining cancer cells.

It only took a few seconds for the actual radiation to be administered, and it didn't make me feel dizzy or overly tired the way chemo had, nor did it have any of chemo's other unpleasant side effects, which was a relief. I was also still going in for my weekly Herceptin infusions and Neupogen shots, which continued to work until mid-July, when my white blood count dropped too low and I had to take a weeklong break from radiation. It was bound to happen with my neutropenia, and I tried not to be discouraged by the setback.

That summer I spent a great deal of time in doctors' offices and medical buildings, rotating on what seemed to be a continuous loop from Dr. Gupta to Dr. Vinciguerra to radiation to Herceptin infusions to Dr. Stills, who had me on an array of supplements to help my body cleanse itself of toxins. I was also having labs twice a week to monitor my white blood count and regular echocardiograms to make sure the Herceptin wasn't damaging my heart.

I tried to stay focused on my own fitness, meditation, and work. I was in the midst of planning Genesis' Annual Fall Legislative Breakfast, to which we invited state and federal officials, members of Congress, and representatives from the autism community. Joanne would be speaking at the breakfast about the challenges of providing ongoing quality services for those with autism in the face of limited funding and increasing costs of care. We had also arranged for parents to tell the stories of their children's self-injurious and aggressive behaviors and how they had needed to make the heartrending decision to place their children in out-of-state facilities because they could no longer care for them. There simply wasn't enough appropriate housing in New York. The work felt vital to me, especially since I was never more aware of the fact that Allan and I wouldn't be alive to take care of Alie and Jamie forever.

———

The boys were having a great summer of races. Alie was closing in on a 20-minute 5K, which we were all excited about, but no one more than Kevin, who loved to see Alie running as fast as he always knew he could.

One day after practice as we all stretched, Kevin laughed and told us how he and Alie had come to some trees at a split in the trail and Alie stopped suddenly and just stood there staring at the tree. They had run from Bethpage State Park to Massapequa Park and back that day, a 13-mile route they hadn't done in a while.

"I couldn't figure out why he stopped or why he was fixated on the tree, and then I remembered that a couple of months ago I'd stopped at that same tree to pee!" Kevin shook his head, smiling. "Alie remembered and stopped on a dime when we got there. I love it when he does that sort of thing. It reminds me not to take him for granted. He's always paying attention."

Another time, Kevin had hid his keys in the woods under some leaves, and when he and Alie got back to his car he realized he'd left them behind. But just as he turned to run back and retrieve them, he saw that Alie had them in his hand. Kevin had laughed then, too. "Alie is keenly observant, which isn't that remarkable in and of itself; it's the fact that he is taking all of this stuff in while looking way off in the distance or jumping up and down seemingly 'out of it.' But he's totally tuned in to what is taking place around him."

Allan and I loved that Kevin delighted in Alie, especially because we knew Alie was far from easy to coach. He was doing better staying behind Kevin, and now on longer runs and races, if Kevin could pace Alie for the first few miles, Alie would lock into that pace and continue to run that same speed for the remainder of the race. But though Alie had stopped swiveling his head in the direction of the car or Kevin's keys or some specific point on the horizon, he now sometimes ran with his eyes pinched shut, or he kept his head cocked ninety degrees to the left or right, running the whole workout or race that way. Kevin would move to whichever side Alie was looking and try to block his view while pointing straight ahead as they ran. These new behaviors would manifest with no warning and would often take months (or longer) to resolve.

————

Allan and Jamie were still enjoying running together, and I couldn't believe that I had ever doubted the logic of Allan taking over Jamie's training. I joined them for most practices, and as we ran down the trail together, I reveled in the fact we were able to spend time together like that. I remembered how I'd spent hours playing backgammon with my dad as a teenager. We played one game after another, him beating me and then me beating him, back and forth. We'd start laughing, and soon we'd be hysterical. I couldn't remember what we were laughing about, but we'd laugh until we cried. Allan and I would never have that kind of relationship with Alie and Jamie. But running with Jamie, watching him slip into his relaxed, forever pace, filled me up in the same way those afternoons with my dad did. I felt, quite simply, at home.

Allan was determined to take over running all of Jamie's races with him, but that summer he had a bad MS flare-up with piercing leg cramps. I'd never seen him in so much pain. He said it felt like he was being repeatedly stabbed with a knife, and not even deep tissue massages helped. The pain seemed to make him more tired than ever, and he had to scale back his running. He couldn't even practice with us most days, and I was so relieved that I had been running and could take Jamie out on my own. I relished those afternoons running with Jamie, and I understood why Allan craved that time with him. Our steps quickly fell into sync, *left right left right*. We didn't need words; the sound of our shoes on the trail bound us to one another.

Jamie also still practiced with Rolling Thunder sometimes and ended up running races with their coaches that summer without any difficult behaviors. We were relieved, but I know Allan was anxious to get back to running with him. He missed the quiet camaraderie that existed between them as they looped through the woods at Bethpage.

Randy and Nancy and I met regularly about Blazing Trails. I had secured a number of sponsors for the race, including Brickwell Cycling as our top sponsor, and they agreed to donate a brand-new Cannondale bike as the grand prize. Randy thought that instead of the typical race t-shirt, we should give away a hooded sweatshirt to all registrants, and I loved the idea, especially since the race would be in early November. Allan and I also solicited vendors to supply energy drinks, and we met with GLIRC and the local police department, who agreed to shut down part of the Long Island Expressway service road where the race would start.

Allan got up early on the weekends and went out to races that the boys weren't running in to hand out Blazing Trails brochures. I drove through Great Neck, putting up posters in the library and local coffee and bagel shops. Whenever the boys had a race, I'd bring a box of brochures and hand them out after the race, asking runners to come and support Genesis and raise awareness of autism, and sometimes after races, Alie and Jamie would walk through the parking lot with me and help me tuck brochures under car windshield wipers. At first they just passed the brochures to me, watching intently as I put them under windshield wipers. But soon they were able to do it themselves as long as Allan and I walked alongside them. Since they both liked to finish a task, they seemed to like how the pile of brochures in their hands got smaller with each car. We often stopped to chat about the race with runners in the parking lot, and I could feel support for it growing.

———

I had been warned of the slow progression of fatigue from radiation, and it had finally caught up to me. By the end of the summer I was exhausted, and the daily drive to Long Island Radiology had grown tiresome. The staff there had been wonderful, but I was ready to be done. Finally, on September 12 I had my last treatment, and I was so relieved. Now I only had my weekly Herceptin infusions.

The next day, Allan was back running with Jamie in the Gary Farley Memorial 5K on the grassy hills and winding roads of Cedar Creek Park in Seaford, Long Island. It was a race in memory of a fallen police officer and there were bagpipes at the starting line. But there was also a loud cannon at the starting line, which none of us expected. Allan didn't realize that he and Jamie were standing right next to it, and when it went off, they both jumped, but Jamie was really scared, yelling loudly. Allan had to put his arm around Jamie and tell him he was safe over and over. Despite that, they had a great race, running a 10-minute pace. And Alie came in second place in his age group, running it in 19:33, a new personal record. Both Alie and Kevin were beaming when they walked up to the podium to get Alie's medal.

———

We were excited but nervous about the upcoming Blazing Trails race. We were hoping for at least 200 runners, which would have been a respectable number for our inaugural race. But in the weeks leading up to the event, we watched the registrations come pouring in. Nancy and her daughter Samantha and son Jonathan were a huge part of that. Jonathan, who was a sophomore at a nearby college, was in a film class and for one of his assignments created a documentary about Alie and Jamie.

He spent weeks filming and editing. He filmed me, Mary, Nancy and Joe, and Alie and Jamie at Genesis. It showed the boys doing a puzzle as Nancy described some of the tools they were using to help them communicate. Jonathan had even met the boys and their therapists out at the stable where they had horseback riding lessons each week. I couldn't believe how well it turned out. I was so touched that Jonathan not only spent the time making the film but that he was able to so clearly capture our lives in it.

Nancy arranged to have it shown in a few of the classes at South, and we took Alie and Jamie there to meet with students, hand out information about autism, and register students to run in or volunteer for the race. An honor class made posters about the race and put them up all over the school. Other students signed up to help with fundraising. Allan and I were touched by the outpouring of support. And their hard work paid off. We ended up with over 800 people registered to run the inaugural Blazing Trails 4-Autism race on November 9.

That morning, we were up early. Allan and I got the boys ready, and we all headed to the Great Neck South campus. The day before, it had poured on us as we lugged boxes of sweatshirts, trophies, and water bottles to the high school gym, and we were praying that it wouldn't rain on race day. But it turned out to be one of the most glorious days of the season. Nancy's husband Martin arranged for Channel 7 Eyewitness News weatherman Jeff Smith to be there at the race broadcasting live, and he marveled at the perfect running weather.

Joe met us at the high school to help with Alie and Jamie while I lined up race trophies and Allan carried in boxes from the truck that GLIRC rented. Race registration was in the school gymnasium, where various vendors had set up booths. We arranged for Rolling Thunder to have a table to recruit new volunteers, and most of the team was there to participate in the race. And many of the staff from Genesis and Eden II were there, some of them handing out information about the school, others getting ready for the run.

When I saw Joanne, I gave her a huge hug. "So what do you think?"

"It's awesome," she said, smiling. "You did an amazing job."

Like everyone at Eden II, Joanne had been spreading the word about the race and she was running it herself. When Joe came over with the boys, she gave them both big hugs, too, and I couldn't help thinking about how far we'd come since that day over 15 years ago when she first came to our house to help us set up our home program. We would never have gotten here without all those early years of ABA.

I think both boys were excited to be back on campus, where they hadn't run since cross-country the year before. Randy and Debbie were going to be running with Jamie, Kevin with Alie, and Allan on his own at a slower pace.

When the gun went off, the runners took off across campus, a wave of bodies moving over the hills, and I thought what a perfect way this was to wrap up a challenging year. I was elated as I walked down to the finish line, which was on the track, to wait for them all to come in. The Long Island band Ready in 10 was playing live, their harmonies and thumping bass and drums filling the air. The lead singer, Sal Nastasi, was also one of Long Island's fastest runners and well-known in the running community, so it was a perfect fit. I held the finish tape for the male and female winners, who finished in 21:55 and 25:01 respectively, and the crowds in the bleachers roared.

There was tons of food at the post-race celebration: Panera bagels, fruit, muffins, energy bars, and Gatorade. Runners and spectators kept coming up and congratulating us on how well the race went, and I gave myself over to the excitement, part of me not believing that we had been able to pull it off with the year that we'd had. But I certainly didn't do it alone. Blazing Trails was a true community effort, and in the end we raised almost $25,000 for Genesis programs.

Before we presented the awards for male and female winners and the top three runners in each age group, we gave a special award to Kevin for his dedication to coaching and the boys. He stood next to me and accepted the award, though I knew he coached for the love of it, not for the recognition. But he made us believe that anything and everything was possible.

———

The year ended on a high note. Though I continued to have weekly Herceptin infusions, my white blood count was holding steady, and Dr. Vinciguerra was pleased with my progress. I was excited about celebrating Hanukkah and Christmas.

As a child I had loved Hanukkah, loved lighting the menorah while my dad recited a prayer or passage from the Torah. Then Edie and I would open the small presents that my parents had chosen for each of the eight nights of the holiday. Sometimes my mom couldn't help herself and she gave us two presents in one night. Then we sang

"Maoz Tzur" and "Dreidel, Dreidel, Dreidel" and ate Mom's delicious potato pancakes with applesauce, and Edie and I stuffed ourselves with Hanukkah gelt.

When Allan and I got married, he wanted a Christmas tree, as well, so I bought a small artificial table-top tree for the living room, and after the boys were born, I'd decorate the mantel with the electric menorah and a garland and stockings for the boys, later hanging from it all the boys' school holiday art projects: snowflakes and dreidels and tiny snowmen.

Each night of Hanukkah that year, we stood with the boys and they took turns switching on the lights of the menorah. "Happy Hanukkah," we said, and they responded with their more garbled version of it. Allan set up the electric trains and the musical Santa Claus, and they watched, riveted, as the trains went round and round while Santa sang "Merry Christmas." Then we handed them their wrapped presents: books and puzzles and music and games. They never asked for anything, of course, so like everything else we guessed what they might like. Sometimes we got it right, other times not. Invariably, a gift that I intended for Alie would end up with Jamie and vice versa. As long as they were happy, it didn't matter.

———

I was looking forward to being done with 2008. The boys were both registered to run the New Year's Day 5K out in Farmingdale, and I decided that I'd run it, as well. What better way to ring in the New Year? I felt ready, and I wanted to start the year off running, a testament to my commitment to myself and my health.

The New Year's course was on the runway of the Republic Airport in Farmingdale, and that morning it was freezing, frigid wind blowing across the open field of runways. My fingers and toes were numb in a few minutes, and the cold air stung my lungs, but I felt invigorated. Allan decided to skip the run so he'd be on hand to corral Alie at the finish line, so I'd be running with Jamie on my own, which I was so looking forward to.

It was a low-key race with only about 200 runners, and while we were waiting for the gun to go off, we spotted Maria, a young Rolling Thunder volunteer who was the same age as Jamie and Alie. She had run with Jamie at team practices a few times, and he really liked her, particularly her swishy blond ponytail. She was planning to run the race on her own, but I asked if she wanted to join us, and she smiled. "Sure!" She was a sweet girl, and I was glad to have her with us. And if I fell behind at all, I knew she'd be able to stick with Jamie.

I held Jamie's hand as we waited for the start, but as soon as the gun went off and we began running, I let go, knowing Jamie would quickly settle into a rhythm next to me, which he did. As we took off together, I felt the thrill that I'm sure the boys and Allan felt at the start of each race—an electric shock of adrenaline that seemed to ripple through the crowd of runners.

As we looped around the airport, across the flat, frozen runways, Maria and Jamie began to inch out ahead of me, and soon I was struggling to keep up. "Slow down, Jamie! Wait for me." Maria and Jamie eased up a bit, but I still had to push it to stay close to them. I was running faster than I did during practices, but somehow I still felt wonderful. I focused on the movement of my warming body and thought of the year ahead, a year of possibilities. I couldn't believe I was in the mix, running with all those people, running with Jamie into a new year, a year free of cancer. My eyes burned, a combination of tears and the jarring cold.

We crossed the finish line four seconds apart: Jamie and Maria in 33:05 and me in 33:09. My lungs felt raw and I was out of breath, but I felt alive. I had just run my first race, and I knew it was just the beginning.

21

I HAD EMBRACED COLD-WEATHER running, which I preferred over running in the heat, and that winter I sometimes ran on my own in addition to accompanying Allan, Kevin, and Alie and Jamie three days a week. It became something I craved. As soon as I was out the door, the things that usually cluttered my mind—schedules, emails, challenges we were having with the boys—seemed to evaporate, and it was just me and the sound of my running shoes on the pavement. When I returned home, my head felt clear, and I was better able to keep the small things in perspective.

The boys were both doing fairly well in school and with their home therapists, but then Alie developed a new obsessive behavior. He could have a normal day at school but then come home and zero in on Allan or me. He'd get this detached look on his face and go for our shoulders, pressing on them really hard, a kind of Vulcan nerve pinch. We hadn't had to do SCIP with Alie for a couple of years, but I worried that it would get that bad again. How could that be when everything had been going so smoothly?

Both Allan and I hoped it wouldn't come to that. We could usually redirect him, but often not until after he'd pressed on one of us. It hurt a lot, his grip sending a dagger of pain out across my shoulder and up the side of my neck. Alie targeted me more often than Allan, probably because Allan could withstand the pain better than I could and wouldn't react. Reacting made it worse. If I cried out, surprised, he'd push even harder. Who knew what was going through his head?

We couldn't figure out how to break the cycle of his obsession, and I began wearing a down vest in the house so it wouldn't hurt so much. I met with Mary and Ruth and the team to discuss strategies. As always, the key was to first determine what caused the behavior, but that wasn't always clear. Then the behavior plan would be to either stop the behavior from starting in the first place or somehow replace it with a more acceptable activity.

We decided that as soon as I saw that look come over Alie, I'd remove myself from the room. Sometimes that helped. If I wasn't there for him to target, he would turn to something else. We weren't certain if the behavior was attention seeking or sensory. Maybe it was both. We gave him weights to lift and stretch bands to pull for tension and to occupy his hands, and we tried to keep him busy all the time. If we could keep him occupied starting and completing tasks he loved, the obsessive thoughts didn't seem to take hold as easily.

But one night in February, he wouldn't leave me alone. He kept coming at me again and again. Each time we were able to redirect him, but only for a few minutes before he was back, reaching for me. Finally, I couldn't take it anymore and went into the bathroom and locked the door. But Alie had followed me, and he was banging on the door, desperate to get in so he could satisfy his compulsion. I could hear him vocalizing, getting louder and louder, working himself into a frenzy. I knew he was probably beginning to sweat out there, wringing his hands and bending his wrists back. I could hear Allan trying to calm him down. "Okay, Alie. It's all done. All done. Come with me, let's go back to your puzzle."

Alie knew what "all done" meant, but he wouldn't let it go. He just kept banging and vocalizing. Each time his fist hit the door, I could feel it in my bones. I knew he didn't really want to hurt me. It was his anxiety that had revved him up, set his OCD in motion. But in that moment none of that mattered. I had locked myself in the bathroom so my son wouldn't hurt me. I sat on the bathroom floor and cried and cried.

This went on for weeks. I wore the vest in the house, and we tried to keep Alie busy with activity schedules, with his therapists, going out with Allan and me. Eventually, thankfully, by the time spring blossomed, it just stopped.

It was amazing that none of these intense behaviors spilled into Alie's running. He was a different person when he was out on the trails with Kevin. He was his most relaxed and joyful self, and he was continuing to get faster. He was consistently taking first place in his age group in races, bringing home medals, trophies, and plaques. He loved going up to the podium and getting his award and having his picture taken. Either Kevin or I would walk with him and prompt him to step onto the stage and position him to face the camera amid loud cheers from the crowd. Then he'd look straight into the camera with his biggest smile, so proud.

They had been running longer and longer distances in practices, and Kevin thought Alie was ready for a half marathon, so we signed him up for the Suffolk Half in early March. Kevin had run it the year before and knew and liked the course, which was an out-and-back down Nicholls Road outside of the Suffolk County Community College. They also had a 5K that morning, which Allan and Jamie would run because they hadn't been running the same long distances in practice. And Allan, though he was feeling strong and hadn't had any more major setbacks, didn't yet feel he was ready for a half marathon.

Race day was misty and chilly. Fog hung in the fields before the start of the race, reminding me of early mornings in the Catskills where my family sometimes vacationed when I was a child. It was such an eerie beauty, as if the clouds had descended to earth and now didn't want to depart.

There were about 300 people running that day, and as they started out, I wished I was running too. But most of the time I still waited on the sidelines at races, holding the cooler full of waters and the running bag with extra sweatshirts, and I didn't mind. I loved to watch the boys fly by, completely in their zones.

Jamie had a great race, coming in third place in his age group. "He did awesome," Allan said, smiling as he gave Jamie a high five. "He probably would have done fine in the half."

"Really?" I said, hugging Jamie and handing him his sweatshirt. "Well let's talk to Kevin about it and figure out a good long race for him."

The half marathon course was two large loops, so Allan and Jamie and I were able to cheer on Alie and Kevin as they headed off on their second loop. Kevin smiled and waved, looking totally relaxed, but Alie was staring straight ahead, in his zone, focused on the finish line. He finished in 1:32:34, a 7:04 pace, winning second place in his age group.

We started thinking about a half marathon for Jamie. Jamie was happily running with either Allan or me or both of us at practices, and he usually raced with Allan but sometimes with Randy or Shanthy, whom we still saw regularly. And he was gliding though race after race at more comfortable paces than his earlier races. Allan and I felt good about the decision we made to slow him down and really attend to his way of communicating what he wanted. He was ready to run longer distances now. Kevin agreed and suggested that both boys run the Hamptons Half Marathon in September.

———

In April, I had my last Herceptin infusion. We had to stop two weeks shy of the full year because of my steadily decreasing white cell count. Dr. Vinciguerra said I could keep going with the Neupogen shots and finish with the last two infusions but that I'd risk infection if my neutrophil level got any lower. I'd been so lucky to avoid any major infections over the year of treatment, and I certainly didn't want to risk it now.

"I think it's okay to stop now," said Dr. Vinciguerra. "You've had the benefit of over 95 percent of the planned infusions."

I agreed to end treatment and was thrilled when the following week my MRI showed I was completely free of cancer. I was so relieved that I wept on the phone with Dr. Vinciguerra. "Thank you so much," I said. "Thank you."

I wanted to do something special to celebrate the end of my treatment and being cancer-free, and I decided that we should celebrate my birthday in July by returning to Virginia Beach. A couple of years earlier, we had started to spend Fourth of July week there, and it had become a tradition to spend my birthday, July 2, watching the waves with the prickling of sun on my skin and seagulls scattering into the blue sky above me. The previous summer we couldn't travel because of my daily radiation and all the additional tests and appointments, but this year I was determined that we'd go back. It would be a celebration of so much more than just turning one year older. I called the Marriott hotel and reserved a one-bedroom suite overlooking the ocean.

————

Later that month Kevin wanted to know if we'd be interested in running the Judi Shesh Memorial 5K in Bay Shore. He had been running it for years with Leslie and often with their nieces, Kaitlin and Sierra. They hadn't known Judi, but she had been about the age of Kevin's sister, Anne, when she died of breast cancer. The run raised awareness about breast cancer and money for research and for organizations that provided comfort and aid to local women fighting breast cancer.

The boys couldn't run it because it was the same weekend as the annual Genesis trip to Shelter Island. For the previous few years, once and sometimes twice a year the boys went on a weekend trip with their classmates. One-to-one school staff kept the students busy with activities all day long, then parties with music and dancing at night. The boys always had a great time, and those weekend trips were also a needed respite for Allan and me. It was the only time that we got away on our own. And though I spent half the time worrying how everything was going with the boys, we knew they were in good hands so I was able to relax and spend time with Allan and our friends.

What better way to celebrate each other and my health than to run this race together? It felt symbolic, and I was grateful for a way to help Kevin and his family honor Anne's memory.

The race began and ended at the YMCA at Bay Shore, looping through Bay Shore and Brightwaters on a scenic route that wound its way toward the water. It was hotter than I would have liked, and I was emotional running among all those people who had been touched in some way by breast cancer. But I was also euphoric. Kevin, Leslie, and Allan all placed in their age groups, and I ran what felt like a solid 5K in 33:36.

———

A month later we headed down to Virginia Beach, which was a seven- to eight-hour car trip from Great Neck. But it was an easy drive. The boys loved being in the car, and I had shown them photos from the last time we had made the trip—the beach, the boardwalk, the hotel pool with its slides and waterfalls—so they knew we were headed somewhere they'd have fun. They settled in with their iPods, each of their heads turned toward their window, taking in the landscape outside. I sat in the front seat, the heat of the sun on my arms and chest. I reached for Allan's hand.

"How are you?" he asked glancing at me.

"Great," I said. "This feels right, doesn't it?"

"It does," he said. "Perfect."

That week was filled with joy. I spent my birthday watching the boys and Allan jump into the white froth of crashing waves. Allan also took the boys into deeper water on his boogie board one at a time. He'd take Alie out for a while, then send him running back to me at the beach chairs. As soon as Alie started toward us, Jamie was up, running toward Allan. They'd switch again and again, until Allan was ready to collapse.

Jamie and Allan ran together along the boardwalk, and I rented a bike so I could ride alongside Alie while he ran. It was the perfect place to get away *and* remain active, which was one of my resolutions. I wanted to be as active and healthy and grounded as I could be, not only because it was good for me but because I loved it.

Each evening we walked into town for dinner, where the boys were bewitched by the lights and music and people. And I reveled in the warm breeze on the boardwalk at night. It felt as if we had returned to a different kind of normal, one in which we dealt with the ongoing challenges of autism and OCD, but in which Allan and I were also carving out time and space for us to be happy and healthy.

For the most part, the boys did really well on the trip, though of course they each developed their fixations and rituals. Standing at the shoreline with waves crashing on his feet, Jamie would go into a mime-like ritual, moving his arms one direction, then lunging forward with one leg, then jumping into the water and out again with the same hand movements. It was like a jerky version of tai chi, and it was actually kind of beautiful, though passersby probably wondered what the hell he was doing, and young children openly stared at him. And Alie became obsessed with the tall hotels that lined the boardwalk. We would be sitting in our beach chairs watching the waves and soon Alie's head would be craned behind him so he could stare at the towering buildings. I kept trying to get him to turn around and face the ocean, which he'd do for a minute or two before slowly rotating his head around again. Eventually I just turned his chair around so he could stare at them without getting a stiff neck. Jamie, Allan, and I faced the ocean, and Alie faced the other direction, lost in the glass and steel and brick that reached toward the blue summer sky. We probably looked ridiculous, but it didn't matter. We were happy.

22

THOUGH WE NEVER BECAME complacent regarding the boys' behaviors, we had become a little complacent about their running because they were both doing so well during training and races. But then one day at the end of July when we were at Brady Park in Massapequa Park near the Massapequa Creek Reserve, one of our worst fears was realized.

Allan was running with Jamie that day and I was biking because it was so hot. Kevin was having Alie do 50-meter hill repeats on the bike path, something they'd done in the past without a problem. Kevin and Alie warmed up, and then Kevin picked a spot at the top of a hill, pointed out the landmarks, and told Alie that he would run up the hill fast, stop right there, then walk back down. Because Alie was so prompt-driven and had such an amazing memory for landscape, he'd always stopped exactly where Kevin told him to stop.

Alie did great on the first two repeats, but on the third one he stopped midway up the hill and looked back at Kevin as if he was waiting for a prompt. So Kevin said, "all the way," and Alie took off up the hill.

But this time Alie didn't come back down. Kevin gave him a few more seconds, then ran up the hill to get Alie, but he was gone.

I've thought of that moment a hundred times, what Kevin must have felt when he got to the top of the hill and Alie had vanished. The sudden panic. The fear. The hammering of his heart in his chest.

Kevin started running down the path calling for Alie. Nothing. And a short way up the path there was a fork. If they'd only run one direction in practice, Kevin would have known which way Alie had gone. But they'd run both ways. In that moment he had to make a decision, and he took the wooded trail to the right. But partway down, he realized that he'd never catch Alie, who had gotten too much of a head start. He ran back to the bike path and headed down toward the parking lot, hoping he'd catch him coming from the other direction.

I had just gotten back from my bike ride and was putting my bike on the back of the car when I saw Kevin running toward me, alone. He was pale even as sweat dripped from his temple.

I was confused. "Where's Alie?"

"He ran off," Kevin said, shaking his head, out of breath. "We were doing hills, and he kept going." He looked stricken.

"What?" I said, my mind slow to make sense of it.

"Alie," Kevin said. "We were doing hills. He ran off. I can't find him."

And just like that my worst nightmare—that one of the boys would run away—was happening. *He ran off. No, no, no.* Images of Alie lost and scared, of Alie hit by a car, of Alie drowned in the creek, flipped through my mind at triple speed.

Kevin was off again, heading toward a trail, running fast.

I picked up the phone and called Allan. "Alie's missing! Come back!" I'm not sure what else I said. What else was there to say? This was not really happening. This could not be happening.

Allan and Jamie were a few miles down the bike path, and Allan spun them around. He had never changed directions suddenly like that, nor did he usually run as fast as they began running back toward the parking lot, so Jamie was scared and began to vocalize loudly. "It's okay, Jamie. It's okay," Allan said over and over again, and luckily Jamie adjusted to the faster pace.

I pulled my bike off the back of the car and then was pedaling as fast as I could, dialing 911 with one hand. When the operator answered I rushed through it all: my son with autism, missing, Brady Park. Send the police now! They wanted me to stay put, but there was no way I could just stand there and wait. I kept biking, calling "Alie! Alie!" But was I even going in the right direction? Which way had he gone? "Alie!"

I stopped everyone I saw. I must have looked crazed. But no one had seen him. There was a major highway just to the north of the park. What if he headed that way? How would we ever catch him?

Allan told me later that he stopped every runner and cyclist they passed, jumping in front of them saying, "You have to help me find my son! He's autistic. He's a runner, and he's lost!"

"What does he look like?" they asked.

Allan pointed to Jamie. "Just like him!"

Soon there were a half dozen bicyclists searching for Alie. They all headed back toward the parking lot, then spread out on different trails. When I think back on that day, the way all those people dropped everything to help us find Alie, my throat tightens with emotion. And I feel sick when I think about how awful Kevin felt, full of dread, as if it had been his fault.

I met Kevin on the path, and he was shaking his head, dripping with sweat. "I'm going to drive along the roads," he said, and he was off again, sprinting toward his car.

I rode up and down the bike path, screaming Alie's name. *No, no, no. Where is he?*

Then the police were there, and I was giving them a description of Alie.

How long was Alie missing? It felt like hours, the heat and our collective fear somehow fusing together to stop time. But in reality, he had only been missing 20 minutes when one of the cyclists Allan had roped into helping us found him on the path, standing exactly where he was supposed to stop and turn around during the hill workout.

I felt awful for not thinking about it earlier. I should have known he'd be there because I knew how his autistic mind worked. Later, we pieced it together. When Kevin said "all the way" to Alie after he paused halfway up the hill, Alie must have thought that Kevin wanted him to run the whole way, "all the way" back to the parking lot. So he ran down the left fork but stopped at some point realizing that he'd gone too far or realizing that Kevin wasn't behind him. He must have turned around and run back, but by that point Kevin had gone down the right fork searching for him. So Alie followed Kevin's original directions: he ran back up the hill and stopped where he had been told to stop. He stopped and just stood there the entire time we were looking for him. When the cyclist found him, he stood next to Alie, talking softly until Allan and Jamie appeared. Kevin arrived a minute later.

When I got to them, I threw down my bike and wept, hugging Alie—Alie who was just standing there; Alie who seemed unfazed, totally fine.

Kevin looked like he was going to pass out, drenched from panic and adrenaline. Not to mention that he'd just sprinted miles, all-out. I knew Kevin felt horrible, and I knew the what-ifs would continue to fire in his brain for days. But this wasn't Kevin's fault. It was Alie. It was autism.

A lot of coaches would have thrown in the towel after that. Who would want to put themselves in that position, assume all of that responsibility? I knew it was a lot to ask, sometimes too much. We wouldn't have blamed Kevin if he'd decided he no longer wanted to coach Alie. But of course he didn't. He loved Alie and Jamie, and he wouldn't give up on them, on us.

I know that day haunted Kevin for a long time, though. And the fear that something like that could happen again probably sucked the joy out of training for a while. But Kevin didn't let that stop him and Alie. The boys were registered for the Hamptons Half Marathon at the end of September, and we had training to do.

———

Allan was nervous about the half marathon. Even though he and Jamie had been running longer distances in practice, he was concerned that he might not be able to finish. What if he had a flare-up just before the race or developed a leg cramp while running?

"You can do it!" Randy told him one day. But she could tell he was still nervous, so she agreed to run it with them for moral support. By this point Randy had run a dozen marathons and countless other races, and she knew Jamie as well as anyone. If Allan had to bow out of the race, she'd have no trouble running it with Jamie. Knowing she'd be running with them seemed to assuage Allan's worries, and he focused on increasing their distance in training.

Because East Hampton was several hours from Great Neck, we all decided to stay nearby at the Ocean Colony in Amagansett the night before the race, and I also reserved rooms for Randy and Kevin and his family.

We all settled into our rooms overlooking the dunes and ocean and then met on the beach. It was a warm and sunny day, and it was relaxing to just sit and chat with Leslie and Kevin. The boys watched the waves, and Kevin flew Mercy over his head, a giggling airplane. When Randy arrived, we all went out for dinner, and Alie and Jamie were on their best behavior, basking in the pre-race rituals of eating pasta and picking up race bibs and arranging their running clothes.

The race started and ended at the Springs School in East Hampton, and it was another beautiful morning. At the start, Kevin and Alie lined up at the front alongside the fastest runners. I snapped a photo in which Alie and Kevin are both smiling broadly. Allan and Jamie and Randy were in the middle of the pack, and I couldn't see them, but I wanted to wish Jamie luck. I moved along the sideline until I saw him, and when he looked up, I threw him a kiss. He smiled and I could tell he vocalized something. I smiled too, grateful that he'd seen me. I knew he didn't know how far he'd be running, but I wanted him to know I was proud of him. It was his first half marathon.

They all had a strong race. Allan and Randy said Jamie was in heaven, skipping the whole way. And Randy and Allan both felt great, as well. They ran it in 2:36:03, a 12-minute pace. Kevin said that Alie had locked into a 6:55 pace early. He came in first in his age group and 21st overall out of over 1,000 runners, running it in 1:30:38. We were all ecstatic.

———

Because the boys had each done well in the half marathon, later that day we talked about how fun it would be to have them run the full marathon there the following year. Kevin thought it would be the perfect first marathon because it was low-key compared to other marathons, and we were already familiar with the course and setup. Kevin was thrilled at the prospect of a marathon, which he hadn't run since he lived in Thailand. He knew Alie could do it—they'd been running 12- to 15-mile practices—and Alie had never once quit in the middle of a run. Allan loved the idea, as well. And though it would be a whole different level of training for him and Jamie, judging from Jamie's performance in the half, they could meet the challenge.

But most marathoners trained six or seven days a week. Some even trained twice a day. Even though we always took the boys on long walks on our non-running days and sometimes Allan and I took them out with our bikes, they still usually only ran three days a week, which is what Kevin could fit in around his work and family schedules. Could they pull off 26.2 miles training three days a week? We'd have to wait and see.

23

WHEN THE BOYS WERE YOUNG, if someone had told me that they would be marathoners, I wouldn't have believed it. Especially Alie, with his years of intense anxiety, self-injury, and aggression, always rushing from one thing to another, nothing holding his attention for long. How could boys who spun and flapped and climbed and screeched ever have the discipline and focus to run 26.2 miles?

It would have seemed impossible.

But as 2009 became 2010 and the boys turned 20, it was clear that they *were* going to become marathoners. Though they were only running three days a week, they were running longer and longer practices. Kevin had done research about the best way to train the boys on three days, and they were doing well on two long runs and one slightly shorter run at a faster pace. Even Allan loved the long distances, heading out on the trail for hours at a time. He incorporated aspects of the Galloway method into his training, alternating running and walking to make sure they could tackle that distance without injury or exhaustion.

It was amazing to me that I had two sons who were not only runners but *really good* runners. I thought back to those early days at the park when, to those nervous, staring parents, I'd said so often, "They're autistic." Over the years, the boys' autism had become such a defining part of who they were. But now, there was something else that defined them. Now I said, "These are my sons. They're runners." And each time, I felt a wave of pride.

———

The Hamptons Marathon that year was at the beginning of October, and just as I had for the half marathon the year before, I arranged for rooms for all of us at Ocean Colony in Amagansett the night before the race.

Kevin knew Alie was ready, but Allan was a little worried about himself and Jamie. Even veteran runners faltered in marathons. This would be their first one, and they had only run up to about 18 miles in practice. But Jamie seemed completely at ease with that distance, settling easily into his forever pace. Allan felt he could do it, and Kevin agreed. But Allan wasn't sure how much farther *he* would be able to run. We talked to Randy, who offered to run the last eight miles of the race with them just in case Allan couldn't finish. Kevin had it all worked out. After he and Alie crossed the finish line, he would drive Randy to mile 18 to wait for Jamie and Allan, and she would jump in and finish the race with them.

In the days leading up to the marathon we checked and double-checked to make sure we had everything we needed: the running cooler, running bag, bagels, the toaster, energy bars, GU energy packs, Allan's running belt, and hydration bottles.

I also had to bring the boys' favorite reinforcers: their iPods for the car ride and for any down time in the hotel room, their favorite snacks, books, and travel puzzles. And because they both excelled as visual learners, I made a social story picture book for them from the half marathon the year before so that they could see the Ocean Colony and the beach and Kevin and Leslie and Mercy with a short description on each page: "We are going to a hotel on the beach." "We will see Kevin and Leslie and Mercy and Randy." "Alie will be running a marathon race with Kevin." "Jamie will be running a marathon race with Daddy and Randy." "We will have fun!"

We had two coolers: a red one for running and races and a blue one for non-running outings such as the beach or walks. We packed up the red one with the usual waters, iced tea, and Gatorade but decided to leave our blue cooler home. We could have used the extra cooler space, but over the years Alie had developed severe OCD around it. Unless we were able to redirect him, he would spend hours sitting on the kitchen floor, arranging the cooler straps. Then he'd stand back and stare at it, only to begin arranging again. Then he would rap the floor with his knuckles. We made sure he knew that the cooler was staying home and let him pack up the running cooler with waters and Gatorade.

Friday morning, we headed out to the Hamptons. It was a perfect fall day, cool but sunny, and as we made our way along the Long Island Expressway, I couldn't help but feel excited. The boys knew we were heading to a race, and as we broke off Sunrise Highway, even if I hadn't shown them the picture book, they probably would have known that we were headed back to the Hamptons.

Allan seemed nervous, and I kept telling him he was going to do great. I had increased my miles over the last year, as well, often running four or five miles during practices, but I couldn't imagine running 26. I kept that to myself, of course, instead reaching for Allan's hand and giving it a squeeze. "You're going to have an amazing race!"

I was looking forward to the beauty of the beach and to staying at the Ocean Colony again, which was surrounded by protected state park land, where the wind whipped over the dunes and carried sand out across the beach. But more than anything, I was looking forward to watching the boys and Allan run their first marathon. I couldn't stop smiling, full of pride and anticipation.

We settled in as we had the year before and spent the afternoon at the beach with Kevin and Leslie and Mercy. It had rained that morning, and it was still cloudy and chilly, but that didn't dampen our spirits. We then met up with Randy and all headed into town to pick up our race packets and have a large pasta dinner. Afterward, Alie arranged his and Allan's and Jamie's running clothes and shoes, and Allan and I got them showered and into bed.

I could hear them tossing and turning in bed, and I knew they were excited about the race, but finally they both settled down and fell asleep.

When I climbed into bed next to Allan, I smiled. "This is so exciting, isn't it?"

"It is," Allan said, but he looked nervous.

"What about you? How do you feel?"

"I know Jamie will be okay, but I hope I can hold up." He rubbed his forehead. "I know the last few miles of a marathon can be brutal."

"You're going to do great. I know it," I said, reaching for his hand. He smiled. "Hope so."

———

Marathon morning, we woke early and had toasted bagels and cream cheese in the room before heading into East Hampton, where the race started and finished, just as the half marathon had the year before. The course was a big loop with a few smaller loops and out-and-backs along the way. It was still dark outside when we arrived at the Springs School, the race headquarters.

Behind the school we met Kevin and Leslie and Mercy, who was in her stroller and looked sleepy but happy. Alie and Jamie were smiling, soaking up the music and people and the pre-race excitement. We took photos, then the boys stretched and Kevin took Alie for a short warm up jog and Allan and Jamie did the same. When they got back, the boys both seemed relaxed and happy, excited to run.

We had about a half hour before start time, so we were all chatting when all of a sudden Alie lunged toward Leslie and Mercy. Allan caught him by the arm and pulled him back toward me. Our eyes met. What was wrong? Alie never acted up before a race.

But Alie was definitely agitated, his anxiety gaining force. He started whining and pulling hard on Allan's sleeve, looking down at Mercy's stroller. Allan and I both looked toward it. What was going on?

That's when we both noticed the cooler under the stroller. It was blue, identical to the one Alie was obsessed with, the one we had intentionally left at home in our pantry. Oh my God. What were the chances? Alie zeroed in on it, thought it was ours, and knew it wasn't where it should be. He had a frenzied look on his face. Allan and I looked at each other. "Fuck," he mouthed. This could derail the whole race.

"Here," he said, passing Alie's hand into my own. "Take Alie away." But it was hard for me to hold on to Alie. He was straining to get the cooler. Luckily Randy was right there, so I passed Jamie's hand to her.

Allan was whispering to Leslie, who looked startled.

Alie had started to sweat and was pulling hard. I knew I had to get him out of there. If he got to that cooler, he'd flip out and start an obsessive ritual that would cost him the start of the race.

Kevin had never seen Alie in the throes of his OCD, and I think both he and Leslie were stunned by how agitated he was.

Finally I pulled on Alie's arm and got him turned in the other direction. "Let's go see what's in these tents," I said, pointing to the vendor tents 10 yards away. I pulled him along with me, though he kept looking over his shoulder, his eyes on the cooler.

When I had gotten Alie out of sight and into one of the vendor tents, Allan grabbed the cooler and hid it under a nearby car. He felt awful hiding their cooler, even though we could come back and get it after the race started.

A few minutes later when we walked back over to everyone, Alie looked all over, toward the stroller, on the ground, searching for the cooler. We kept distracting him and finally just repeated over and over, "Nope, the cooler's gone. No more cooler. We're getting ready to run." Would he perseverate on this? What if he ran off at the start of the race to look for it? I remembered his head-swiveling phase, when he'd run with his head pointed in the direction of the car or wherever Kevin had left his keys. What if he started up with that again today?

But then Kevin stepped in and took Alie's hand. "Come on Alie, let's go run a marathon!" Alie smiled distractedly, but off they went, walking hand in hand to the start as we followed behind.

Randy shook her head, smiling. "Thank God running is such a powerful reinforcer for him."

"I know," I said, relieved.

But I was still nervous as we made our way to the starting line. Would Alie settle into race mode or would the cooler incident disrupt his run? I needn't have worried. When I saw Kevin and Alie standing in the crowd right up front with the elites, I could see Alie was in his element: focused, ready to run.

By that point, the sun had risen, and I could tell it was going to be a gorgeous day, the perfect day for the boys' first marathon. Leslie, Mercy, Randy, and I stood together as we waited for the gun to go off. I grabbed Randy's arm. "Do you think they're going to be okay?"

"They're going to do great!" Randy laughed.

Leslie smiled and said the same thing. "They've worked so hard for this!"

"You're right," I said, smiling. They had, and I knew they'd do it.

When the gun went off, we cheered into the cool fall air. "I can't believe this," I said, full of wonder. "I can't believe they're running a marathon!"

Randy laughed. "I know!"

Our plan was to cheer for them at mile six, then again at 22, then head to the finish line. Because the race was laid out the way it was, we only had to walk a couple of miles to be able to see them in three places on the course.

At mile six we stood in the bright sun, watching for Kevin and Alie. When we saw them, we screamed their names and jumped up and down. I felt like a little kid. Randy told all the other spectators standing near us about Alie and his autism, so they were cheering for him, too. Both Kevin and Alie looked amazing. Alie was focused straight ahead and barely looked at us, but Kevin gave us a thumbs up and a big smile as he grabbed the energy drink concoction that Leslie held out to him as he ran by. "He's doing great so far!"

Then we waited for Jamie and Allan, who also looked strong. We screamed their names and Allan smiled and waved. Jamie had clearly settled into his carefree forever pace, a distant smile on his face.

We had retrieved the cooler after the race started, and now we joked about it. "That was your crash course in autism," Randy said, smiling at Leslie. We all laughed.

Mile 22 was the turn before the last loop and a short out-and-back along the shore; then, they'd be headed to the finish line. We screamed for Kevin and Alie again there, and they still both looked strong, Alie totally focused, in his Zen place. We had less than a half hour to walk back to the finish line, and I was nervous about getting back in time to video them coming in. But Leslie and Randy laughed off my worries. "Of course we'll be back before they finish. Don't worry."

We walked quickly back to the finish line, where we stood on the grass at the side of the course. The sun was bright and the crowd was cheering loudly for the runners coming in. As I took it all in, I couldn't believe that they were really doing it, that my sons with such severe autism were running a marathon.

I checked my watch. When Kevin and Alie passed us they were running about a 7:45 pace, but I didn't know if they'd be able to sustain that all the way to the end. Randy ran down to the bend in the road so she could see them coming and give me the sign to start filming, and suddenly I looked over at her, and she was yelling, "He's coming! Alie's coming!"

And there he was, flying, his arms low and fast, telescoped on the finish line. Leslie and other people around us were screaming his name and I was too, my throat tight, my eyes full of tears. "Go, Alie! Go!" He did it!

Randy had jumped into the race, running on the sidelines, yelling after him, "Go! Go! Go!"

Kevin ran by a few seconds later, and he looked like he was struggling. "Go, Kevin!" we yelled.

"Yikes," said Leslie, "He looks like he's in pain."

"I hope he's okay," I said, and we made our way to the finish area.

When I found Alie, he was smiling with a race medal around his neck. I gave him a tight hug and high fives. "Alie, you're amazing. I'm so proud of you!" He'd finished in 3:27:36, a 7:56 pace. And, we'd later learn, first in his age group.

Randy was laughing. "You'll never guess what just happened," she said, shaking her head.

"What?"

"When Alie crossed the finish line he was just standing there, looking up at the sky smiling, and as a volunteer slipped a medal over his neck, he thought Alie looked a little delirious." Randy laughed. "When I came up to him he was asking Alie who the president was, and because Alie couldn't answer, they thought he had heat stroke. Ha! I told them he had autism and had just run an amazing race!"

I laughed. It wouldn't be the first time that happened after the end of a long race.

Then we saw Kevin, who was lying down on the pavement, his hands on his face.

"Are you okay?"

"I just bonked," he said. "I kept cramping, and I had to keep stopping us."

"Oh no," I said, holding Alie's hand in mine. "Are you going to be okay?"

Kevin insisted he was, that he just felt bad about holding Alie back. But Alie clearly didn't mind. He was beaming. He didn't even look winded.

Kevin drank some water and Leslie massaged his legs. He stretched, and then we piled into his car. I held Alie's hand as he sat quietly next to me, a smile frozen on his face. We dropped Randy at mile 18, and then drove back to wait for Jamie and Allan. As I stood there with Kevin, Alie, Leslie, and Mercy, I was flooded with gratitude: for running, for the amazing coaches and teachers that had come into our lives, for Allan and the boys. This was the life we were living. It wasn't an easy one and I knew it never would be, but it was my life and I was determined to live it as fully and with as much joy as I could.

I put my arm around Alie. "I love you, Alie."

"Ah o ooh," Alie said, smiling distantly, watching the runners come in.

I leaned into him, resting my head on his shoulder, the shoulder of my marathon son.

———

Over an hour later, we watched them turn the corner: Allan, Randy, and Jamie running side by side. They did it! They had run a steady race, and Jamie looked elated, skipping into the air as he crossed the finish line in 6:13:41. "Go, Jamie! Yay!" Both Allan and Randy waved, smiling. My heart was full.

We made our way to the finish line again, Alie's hand in my own.

When we found Allan and Randy and Jamie, they were all beaming. I squeezed Jamie tight and kissed Allan. I couldn't believe my sons had just run a marathon! And I was so proud of Allan, as well. I knew how much he'd wanted to finish with Jamie, and he did it! I choked back my tears, basking in what they had just accomplished, rejoicing in how far they'd come—in how far we'd all come.

EPILOGUE

SINCE THAT FIRST RACE IN 2006, my sons have run almost 150 races, including nine marathons. They've had the support from Achilles International, the Boston Athletic Association, and always Rolling Thunder. They've run in countless races to raise awareness of autism, and I wish I could say that was it; that our lives had been uneventful since the boys crossed all those finish lines. But, of course, that wouldn't be true.

Some of our biggest challenges in recent years have been with Jamie, who, though he'd always been extremely low functioning, was always our happy-go-lucky son, the one who for years would go along with just about anything, who ran for the sheer joy of it. But in early 2011, Jamie began to withdraw and show signs of increased anxiety, tensing up with any loud noise, often saying "No, no," as if he was scared. We had to begin prompting him to do things that he had done independently for years, like eating and getting dressed. We couldn't figure it out, and it felt as if we were watching him disappear before our eyes, just as we'd watched autism take hold of him and Alie all those years ago.

He developed anxiety around school, becoming overly sensitive to other students' behaviors, and he began to move in slow motion. What used to take him 45 minutes now took two hours. When he put on his socks, he would freeze, his foot poised in the air for several minutes. If we tried to rush him, he'd blow up, banging his fist on the table. He began biting his hands and even started having bathroom accidents. Allan and I were at a loss, and it was heartbreaking to watch our sweet boy transform.

We later learned that Jamie had developed catatonia, a chronic condition that occurs in approximately 15 percent of adolescents who have autism. Catatonia shares some of the symptoms of autism, but the key distinctions are a "marked change in behavior and no operant cause for self-injurious behavior." Jamie was formally diagnosed in 2012, when we took him to see Dr. Lee Wachtel at the Kennedy Krieger Institute in Baltimore, Maryland. He's gotten much better as a result of medication paired with a complex behavior plan supervised by Mary McDonald as our consultant and Jamie O'Brien, his behavior therapist. But trauma and loud noises always set him back.

It took us months and months to deal with the aftermath of the 2013 Boston Marathon bombing. Both Alie and Jamie ran the Boston Marathon that year. Amazingly, Alie finished in 3:23:22, the exact time, down to the second, of his second Hamptons Marathon. He'd run it with Kevin as well as Stephen, one of our amazing race guides, and as usual he was beaming at the finish line. Kevin said he could have kept going and going.

I was sitting in the front row of the grandstands at the finish line with Stephen's wife, Danielle, and their two children, cheering as they flew by us. Then we went to the family meeting area to celebrate with them and take pictures before heading to our hotel, The Westin Copley Place, to get Alie's sweatshirt. After that, we were going back to the finish line to watch for Jamie and Allan and Katie, one of our former home therapists who was also one of Jamie's race guides.

From our hotel room, we heard the bombs explode. They detonated directly across from where we had been sitting, and if Alie had run the race the same pace he had the year before, I would have been there with Danielle and her children when it happened. I shudder to think about that day, about what would have happened to us if we had gone back to the grandstands. My heart goes out everyone who was so tragically injured and to the families of those who were killed.

We were terrified, especially since I couldn't get ahold of Allan, who was still in the race with Jamie and Katie. Alie was distressed, pulling on my arm, wanting to return to the finish line, which of course we couldn't do. Allan finally texted that he and Jamie had been pulled off the course at mile 22 and had been taken to a church in lockdown. But everyone was screaming and crying, distraught, and Jamie's eyes were wide; he was traumatized, unable to process what was happening. On the car ride home the next day, we could barely talk because Jamie wanted absolute silence, and for months afterward he was jumpier, had trouble sleeping, and became nervous in crowds.

Slowly, Jamie began to recover and started running races and increasing his distance again. But the 2013 New York City Marathon—his first marathon since Boston—was brutal. He started out strong, but then at mile 8, someone blew a horn near his face as he ran by, and he lost it. It took Allan an hour to settle him down enough so he could continue running. They had to take it slow. It was such a long race—the longest race he'd had. But he finished, and when they crossed the finish line at 7:58:16, he was smiling. It was a triumph.

Alie continues to suffer with intense anxiety and OCD, but we manage on a day-to-day basis, trying to divert any new obsessions that emerge. But we know there will always be another one around the corner. For both Alie and Jamie, their inability to communicate, to tell us how they feel and what they want and need, is one of the most difficult challenges we live with every day.

In addition to the challenges that we've grown to expect, we've also celebrated a lot in recent years. I have been cancer-free for six years. I'm still practicing self-care, and though I sometimes need reminders if I slip into old habits, mostly I remember to take time out for myself. I'm running and biking several times a week and I've run dozens of races on my own and with Jamie. My goal is to run my first half marathon in 2015. I can't imagine living any other way now.

At the age of 20, the boys were able to walk in the Great Neck South High graduation ceremony in June of 2011, the year they graduated from the Genesis school and transitioned into the Genesis Day Habilitation program. As Alie and Jamie walked across the stage with their therapists to receive their high school diplomas amid deafening cheers, I wept.

I was the race director for the Blazing Trails 4-Autism race for three more years, and we continued to draw huge numbers of participants and raise awareness of autism and money for Genesis. In 2012, I passed off the coordination of the race to the development coordinator at Genesis, but it continues to be one of our favorite annual races.

My dad had a philosophy on life: "Learn from the past, live for the present, and look to the future." Allan and I have learned to live that way. The future holds many unknowns, of course, as it does for everyone, and my sons' future is always on my mind. I continue to advocate for more funding and more services for individuals with autism, especially those who, like Alie and Jamie, have low functioning autism with severe behavioral challenges. For the rest of their lives they will need care—24 hours a day, 7 days a week—with skilled behavior therapists who know how to manage their always-changing behaviors. We've spent hours on planning committees, trying to guarantee the proper housing and care for them into the future when Allan and I won't be here to take care of them, to nurture their joy and keep them safe. We haven't found the right solution yet, but we will. I have to believe that.

What's amazing to me as I think back on our lives and on these recent years is that for us, running began as something the boys could do to burn their excess energy, to calm them down. But over the years it's something that's brought our family closer together and, most importantly, brought us all joy.

Alie continues to progress as a runner, getting faster and faster with seemingly unlimited potential, and we're so grateful that Kevin still coaches him three days a week. In the 2013 New York City Marathon, Alie ran his personal record, 3:14:36. Incredibly, each mile was faster than the last, and he was the first of all the American and International Achilles Runners to finish the race. Alie can sense the finish line. Who knows how—maybe it's the music and excitement or the other runners around him picking up the pace. But it's as if he's visualizing the finish line, and he always kicks it up a notch, always finishes strong.

He's no longer that wild colt of a teenager who was impossible to pace. "We've been running for so many years now," says Kevin. "There was no epiphany, just a lot of trial and error to figure out what would work for him. But he's morphed into this person who can tell what kind of workout we're going to do—fast, medium, or slow—by what shoes I'm wearing. And now when we're running, if he's too far ahead of me—if he can no longer hear my footsteps—he'll look back and wait for me to say something, and I'll say 'Good waiting, Alie.'"

Jamie, now more than ever, loves to loop through wooded trails or run on a bike path at a slower pace, his forever pace, and either Allan or I, or both of us, run with him. Just the other day, I took Jamie out to Bethpage State Park, and we headed out on the bike path together. Yellow leaves glowed bright in the afternoon sun, and the air was crisp—my favorite running weather. I could feel Jamie settle into his rhythm, a hush descending over him. I don't know what was going through his head—I never will—but I know he was at peace, happy in that moment. And so was I.

ACKNOWLEDGMENTS

THERE ARE SO MANY PEOPLE in my life that have left an imprint on my heart, to whom I am so grateful. Thank you for inspiring me to share my story with the world. But most of all, thank you for supporting us and loving Alex and Jamie.

My dear friends, you have always been there for me. From the beginning of Alie and Jamie's diagnosis, having your shoulder to lean on helped me navigate this journey and enabled me to find my way. What started out as professional relationships turned into friendships that I cherish every day. Thank you to Ruth Donlin, Randy Horowitz, Mary McDonald, and Joanne Gerenser for your friendship and support, and especially for the many hours you spent guiding me through the complexities of autism. You embraced my sons and taught me the skills I needed to enrich their lives. To my friends Brenda Coleman, Nancy Philips, Danielle Dalton, Susan Timler, and Linda Meyer, thank you for caring and loving the boys the way you do, and for cheering them on through the years.

To my loving family, both Allan's and mine. You bring sunshine to our world, and your unconditional love for Alie and Jamie warms my heart. To Edie, my sister, thank you for your love and understanding and for sharing all your memories and recollections of our childhood years together. Thank you Cheri for your warmth and being here when I needed you most.

To my friend Bob Pidkameny, thank you for your kindness and concern for Alie and Jamie and their future. I am so appreciative of the countless hours you devoted to designing potential creative housing opportunities to meet their needs and the needs of the autism community on Long Island.

Thank you to Theresa, Marjorie, and Barbara for the many years you spent with our family, cooking your delicious meals and caring so much for my sons.

To all of our many home therapists over the years, thank you for your dedication and commitment to Alie and Jamie, and for your patience, love, and devotion. They are so lucky to have all of you in their lives.

We are grateful to all the organizations that have supported Alie and Jamie over the years. A huge thank you to the following organizations and their staff: The Eden II Genesis Programs, Rolling Thunder Running Club, Achilles International, Association for Science in Autism Treatment (ASAT), Organization for Autism Research (OAR), Autism Speaks, The Boston Athletic Association, New York Road Runners, Greater Long Island Running Club, My Shine Therapeutic Riding Program, the Great Neck School District, Long Island Advocacy Center, NY Self-Determination Coalition (NYSELFD), Lee Stockner's Music Box Method, Long Island Developmental Disabilities State Office, SCO Family of Services, Life Services, Independent Support Services (ISS), Omni Publicity, Pacebands, Elija School and Foundation, EJ Autism Foundation, Alpine Learning Group, Autism New Jersey, and Nassau Suffolk Services for Autism (NSSA).

There have been many doctors who have cared for my family and me over the years. I am especially grateful to Dr. Karen Kostroff, Dr. Vincent Vinciguerra, Dr. Lee Watchel, Dr. Marcia Bergtraum, Dr. Arun Gupta, Dr. Sharon Stills, and Dr. Jane Perr. Thank you for your patience, your knowledge, your sensitivity, and your kindness.

I am most grateful to the following people and media outlets that have shared our story so eloquently: Corey Kilgannon, the *New York*

Times; Suzanne Yeo and Linzie Janis, ABC's *Good Morning America*, ABC's *World News Tonight with David Muir*; David Willey, *Runners World Magazine*; *Cosmopolitan*; Al Jazeera; *Newsday*; *The Southampton Press* and *The East Hampton Press*; *Anton Community Newspapers*; the *Boston Herald*; Kennedy Krieger Institute's *Potential* Magazine; *USA Today*; and Verizon Fios. Thank you for seeing my sons as the amazing runners they are.

My sons are able to compete in races because of the dedication and commitment of several very special individuals. Each time they stand on that starting line next to Alie or Jamie, they are taking on a huge responsibility, yet they do so enthusiastically and selflessly. I have the deepest appreciation for Alie and Jamie's race guides: Stephen Dalton, Matt Connors, Katie Raab-Reed, Shanthy Hughes, Philip Lang, Robert Votruba, Spencer Gallop, John Jones, James Kennedy, Mike Kelly, Rick Lipsey, and all the other Rolling Thunder volunteers who have run with my sons through the years.

The person I am most deeply appreciative of and have the most gratitude for is Kevin McDermott. Kevin has the biggest heart of anyone I know. He is passionate, honest, and so generous with the time he has so willingly devoted to Alie and Jamie. We are so fortunate that you entered our lives, Kevin, and are thankful every day for your infectious enthusiasm, knowledge, incredible talent, and patience. And most of all, I am grateful for the friendship we have developed with you, Leslie, and your lovely family. Leslie, I am so appreciative to you for graciously sharing your husband each week to run with my family.

Thank you to my agent, Chris Park of Foundry Literary and Media, for seeing the potential in my story and believing in its power.

Kate Hopper, thank you for your talent and expertise and for working so zealously with me in retelling my story. You have become a special friend. And to Bonnie J. Rough, thank you for your attentive reading and editorial suggestions.

To Triumph Books: Tom Bast, Noah Amstadter, Adam Motin, Michelle Bruton, Tom Galvin, Andrea Baird, Josh Williams, Emily Oprins, and Bill Ames. Thank you so much for believing in me and my story and for sharing my passion. I am forever grateful for your enthusiasm and support in bringing *Silent Running* to fruition.

To my parents, Frances and Ingram. I will always treasure your smiles, your laughter, your kindness and generosity, your determination, and your love. Thank you for your wisdom and for the life lessons you taught me and for always seeing the beauty within. You are forever in my heart.

To my husband Allan, my soulmate, best friend, lover, and confidant. Thank you for our cherished memories and for helping me to share our intimate story.

And finally, to my beautiful sons, Alie and Jamie. In my heart I believe that somehow you know how much I love and admire you. You are the loves of my life and I am truly blessed to be your mother.